W9-CYY-796

Diseases of the Salivary Glands
Including Dry Mouth and Sjögren's Syndrome

Springer
Berlin
Heidelberg
New York
Barcelona
Budapest
Hong Kong
London
Milan
Paris
Santa Clara
Singapore
Tokyo

Isaäc van der Waal

Diseases of the Salivary Glands Including Dry Mouth and Sjögren's Syndrome

Diagnosis and Treatment

With Collaboration of Leo M. Sreebny

With 58 Figures and 12 Tables

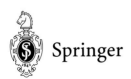 Springer

Prof. Dr. Isaäc van der Waal
University Hospital
Dept. of Oral & Maxillofacial Surgery/Pathology
P.O. Box 7057
1007 MB Amsterdam, The Netherlands

Prof. Dr. Leo Sreebny
State University of New York at Stony Brook
School of Dental Medicine
Dept. of Oral Biol. & Pathol.
and Dept. of Family Medicine
Stony Brook, NY 11794-8702, USA

ISBN 3-540-61380-3 Springer-Verlag Berlin Heidelberg New York

Library of Congress Cataloging-in-Publication Data. Waal, Isaäc van der, 1943– Diseases of the salivary glands including dry mouth and Sjögren's syndrome: diagnosis and treatment/Isaäc van der Waal; with collaboration of Leo M. Sreebny. p. cm. Includes bibliographical references and index. ISBN 3-540-61380-3 (hardcover: alk. paper) 1. Salivary glands—Diseases. I. Sreebny, Leo M. (Leo Morris), 1922– . II. Title. [DNLM: 1. Salivary Gland Diseases—diagnosis. 2. Salivary Gland Diseases—therapy. WI 230 W111d 1996] RC815.5.W32 1996 616.3′16—dc20 DNLM/DLC for Library of Congress 96-22209

© Springer-Verlag Berlin Heidelberg 1997
Printed in Germany

Cover Design: Design & Production GmbH, Heidelberg

Typesetting: Best-set Typesetter Ltd., Hong Kong

SPIN: 10522664   23/3134/SPS – 5 4 3 2 1 0 – Printed on acid-free paper

Preface

Saliva has multiple functions in protecting the integrity of the oral mucosa: it participates in clearing the oral cavity of food residue, debris, and bacteria; it buffers to some extent the deleterious effects of strong acids and bases; it provides the ions needed to remineralize the teeth; and it has antibacterial, antifungal, and antiviral capacity. In addition, components of saliva facilitate the motor functions of chewing, swallowing, and speaking and also have sensory and chemosensory functions in the oral cavity. Thus saliva plays an important role in many respects.

Diseases of the salivary glands occur with varying frequency in both the major and the minor salivary glands. In arriving at a correct diagnosis, history and clinical findings are important to a greater or lesser extent. In addition, a large number of investigative techniques are available, such as sialometry, sialochemistry, sialography, computed tomography, magnetic resonance imaging, scintigraphy, ultrasonography, aspiration cytology, and histological examination. In discussing the various diseases of the salivary glands, these diagnostic tools will be briefly commented on, thus assisting clinicians in the management of patients.

This monograph was primarily written for use in the daily practice of all medical and dental professionals involved in the diagnosis and treatment of the various salivary gland diseases, including dry mouth and Sjögren's syndrome. Furthermore, attention has been paid to the possible involvement of the salivary glands in systemic diseases.

The text of Chap. 1 is largely based, with permission, on a monograph prepared by a Working Group of the Commission on Oral Health, Research and Epidemiology, Fédération Dentaire International, published in a supplement of the *International Dental Journal* in 1992 (vol. 42 suppl. 2, pp. 291–304). The authority of Professor

Leo M. Sreebny, who chaired the FDI Working Group, is fully acknowledged.

The close collaboration with Professor Gordon B. Snow, head of the Department of Otolaryngology at the University Hospital, Vrije Universiteit, Amsterdam, is gratefully acknowledged. Much of the experience reflected in this book with regard to salivary gland neo-plasms is the result of numerous discussions with him. Furthermore, I am indebted to professor B. Nauntofte from the Department of Oral Function and Physiology, School of Dentistry, Faculty of Health Sciences, University of Copenhagen, Denmark, for her critical com-ments and suggestions for Chaps. 1 and 3. Dr. Henk Kraaijenhagen and Dr. Graham Putnam (United Kingdom) have critically reviewed the manuscript, resulting in several improvements.

I would like to thank Mrs. Dini Chevalking for her dedication during the preparation of the manuscript and Mr. G.J. Oskam and Mr. J.T. van Veldhuisen for their help with photography.

Amsterdam, The Netherlands   I. van der Waal
July 1996

Contents

1 Dry Mouth and Hypersalivation

1.1 Introduction

The mixed oral fluids, referred to as "whole" saliva, mainly consist of secretions from the major and minor salivary glands. In addition, whole saliva contains a number of constituents of nonsalivary origin, such as bacteria, desquamated epithelial cells, crevicular fluid, and food debris.

Saliva is secreted in response to neutrotransmitter stimuli. During most of the day, neurotransmitter release is low and a basal or "unstimulated" flow occurs. During food consumption, in response to gustatory and masticatory stimuli, there is a marked release of neurotransmitters and secretion is stimulated. Basal salivary flow is considered to be a protective secretion, while the large, stimulated flow is needed to facilitate ingestive processes (food bolus formation and swallowing) and communication (Table 1.1). Patients with a total lack of salivary flow rarely have normal-appearing oral mucosa [45].

A number of factors influence the composition of whole saliva, in particular the source, collection method, and degree of stimulation. In response to stimulation, saliva output may increase manifold, with significant changes in consistency and in the concentration of many of its constituents [7].

Several techniques may be used to measure salivary gland function, including sialometry, scintigraphy, sialography, and sialochemistry.

1.2 Composition of Saliva

About 99% of saliva is water. The remaining 1% consists for the most part of large organic molecules, e.g., proteins, glycoproteins, and lipids; small organic molecules, e.g., glucose and urea; and electrolytes, chiefly sodium, calcium, chloride, and phosphates. Most of the organic molecules are produced by the acinar cells, some are synthesized in the ducts, and some are transported into the saliva from the blood. A list of salivary constituents in alphabetical order, subdivided into proteins, small organic molecules, and electrolytes is given in Table 1.2.

Sialochemistry assays the concentration of various salivary constituents, e.g., the levels of electrolytes or proteins and the presence of drugs and hormones. It requires a special laboratory, such as is normally associated with oral biology units in dental schools, and is best performed on saliva from individual salivary glands.

The *parotid* glands have serous acinar cells and produce a proteinaceous, watery secretion; the secretion from the *sublingual* glands is mucous and hence more viscous. The *submandibular* glands have both serous and mucous acinar cells and produce saliva with a lower protein content and a higher viscosity than the parotid glands. The *minor* salivary glands, distributed throughout the oral cavity, are purely mucous glands.

As the salivary flow rate increases, the concentrations of proteins, sodium, chloride, and bicarbonate rise, while the levels of phosphate and magnesium fall.

Table 1.1. The major functions of saliva [35]

Function	Salivary components involved
Protective functions	
Lubrication	Mucins, proline-rich glycoproteins; water
Antimicrobial	Salivary proteins: lysozyme, lactoferrin, lactoperoxidase, mucins, cystatins, histatins, secretory IgA; proline-rich glycoproteins
Mucosal integrity	Mucins, electrolytes, water
Lavage/cleansing	Water
Buffering	Bicarbonate, phosphate ions
Remineralization	Calcium, phosphate, statherin, anionic proline-rich proteins
Food- and speech-related functions	
Food preparation	Water, mucins
Digestion	Amylases, lipase, ribonuclease, proteases, water, mucins
Taste	Water, gustin
Speech	Water, mucins

Table 1.2. Salivary constituents [35]

Proteins	Small organic molecules	Electrolytes
Albumin	Creatinine	Ammonia
Amylase	Glucose	Bicarbonate
β-Glucuronidase	Lipids	Calcium
Carbohydrases	Nitrogen	Chloride
Cystatins	Sialic acid	Fluoride
Epidermal growth factor	Urea	Iodide
Esterases	Uric acid	Magnesium
Fibronectin		Nonspecific buffers
Gustin		Phosphates
Histatins		Potassium
IgA		Sodium
IgG		Sulfates
IgM		Thiocyanate
Kallikrein		
Lactoferrin		
Lipase		
Lactic dehydrogenase		
Lysozyme		
Mucins		
Nerve growth factor		
Parotid aggregins		
Peptidases		
Phosphatases		
Proline-rich proteins		
Ribonucleases		
Salivary peroxidases		
Secretory component		
Secretory IgA		
Serum proteins (trace)		
Tyrosine-rich proteins		
Vitamin-binding proteins		

Ig, immunoglobulin.

1.3 Collection of Saliva and Measurement of Flow Rate

Sialometry measures the flow rate of saliva. The techniques associated with it can readily be performed in the dental or medical office. The purpose and method of the procedure should be explained to the patient beforehand.

Saliva should be collected about 1.5–2h after eating or after overnight fasting. Patients should be instructed to do nothing that might stimulate the flow of saliva prior to collection. This prohibition includes mastication of anything (e.g. food, chewing gum, candy), smoking, toothbrushing, mouthwashes, and drinking. The test should be conducted in a quiet area.

Whole saliva may be collected and measured by a variety of volumetric and gravimetric techniques, including draining (drooling), spitting, suction, and swab. The volumetric methods to be described, especially a combination of the drooling and spitting techniques, are easily performed in the dental or medical office. Resting salivary flow rates are roughly equivalent for draining, spitting, suction, and swab collection techniques, but the swab technique is less reliable [27].

Two measuring devices may be employed: a "sialometer" or any finely calibrated measuring cylinder. The sialometer is a specially constructed, reusable, commercially available device, which enables the practitioner to collect both resting and stimulated saliva in a single vessel. Alternatively, two measuring cylinders of about 12 ml in volume, calibrated to no less than 0.1 ml, and two funnels are needed. These can generally be obtained from chemical supply houses.

In a recent paper, a simplified method was proposed in which whole saliva, either stimulated or unstimulated, is sampled with small gauzes inserted in the sublingual groove and left in place for a set number of minutes; the gauzes are then weighed [19]. The reliability of this method has still to be confirmed.

To obtain mean flow rates, at least two tests should be performed, at about the same time of the day, on two different days. If the patient's baseline has been established earlier, the values obtained can be used as a comparative indicator of the patient's present salivary status. If the baseline is not known, as is usually the case, the flow rates have to be compared with the pertinent population standards. As with any test, the results should be interpreted in the light of the patient's history, the presence of any signs of disease, and the results of other tests.

1.3.1 Collection of Whole Saliva

1.3.1.1 Unstimulated (Resting) Whole Saliva

The patient is seated, head slightly down, and is asked not to swallow or move his or her tongue or lips during the collecting period. The saliva is allowed to accumulate in the mouth for 2 min – some prefer longer periods – and he or she is then asked to spit the accumulated saliva into the receiving vessel. This procedure is performed twice more for a total of 6 min. The flow rate, expressed as ml/min, is the total volume of saliva collected divided by 6.

1.3.1.2 Stimulated Whole Saliva

The most important stimuli to salivation are mastication and gustatory stimuli. Chewing a flavorless bolus such as paraffin wax leads to an increase in saliva flow of about threefold; gustatory stimuli may cause a tenfold increase in saliva flow [7].

Paraffin Method (Masticatory Stimulus). The patient is asked to hold a piece of paraffin wax in his or her mouth until it becomes soft (about 30 s) and then to swallow the saliva which has collected in the mouth. The patient is then asked to chew the piece of wax in his or her usual manner of chewing for exactly 2 min and then to expectorate the accumulated saliva into the receiving vessel. The procedure is repeated twice more. The volume of saliva is read off the vessel and flow is expressed as ml/min.

Citric Acid Method (Gustatory Stimulus). A 2% solution of citric acid (made up at a local pharmacy) is swabbed on to the laterodorsal surface of the tongue every 30 s for a period of 2 min. The saliva is then expectorated into the receiving vessel. As in the paraffin method, the whole procedure is repeated twice more, for a total time of 6 min. As before, the flow is expressed as ml/min.

1.3.2 Collection of Saliva from the Individual Salivary Glands

Parotid saliva is usually obtained using a modified, two-chambered Carlson-Crittenden collector [9]. The inner chamber is placed over the orifice of Stensen's duct; the outer chamber is attached, via thin tubing, to a rubber bulb which, when compressed, creates a slight negative pressure and permits the device to adhere to the surrounding mucosa. This device makes it possible to collect pure parotid saliva in a noninvasive manner (Fig. 1.1).

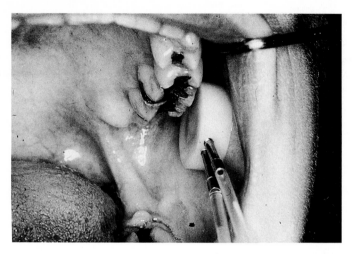

Fig. 1.1. Collection of parotid saliva. (Courtesy of Dr. L.F.E. Michels, Netherlands)

In order to collect only *submandibular/sublingual* saliva, the region of Wharton's ducts should be isolated with gauze from the rest of the mouth, particularly from the orifices of Stensen's ducts. The saliva, resting or stimulated, which has collected during a given time is aspirated with a plastic micropipette. The flow rate is expressed as ml/min per pairs of submandibular/sublingual glands.

Saliva may be obtained from the *minor salivary glands* of the lower lip or the palate. The minor glands are dried and isolated with gauze or cotton rolls. After 2 min for resting saliva, the fluid which is present at the orifice of one or more of these glands is adsorbed on to filter strips; the filter strips are then placed into a device which electronically reads the volume of fluid on each strip. For stimulated minor gland saliva, the tongue is swabbed with a 2% citric acid solution, as described above. The results are expressed as µl/min. Since the number of glands and the area sampled vary, the flow rate is semiquantitative.

1.3.3 Flow Rate of Saliva

There have been many studies of salivary flow rates in individuals presumed to be healthy from different countries. The resting flow rate for whole saliva averages about 0.3–0.4 ml/min; flow stimulated by paraffin chewing averages 1–2 ml/min (Table 1.3). Unstimulated whole salivary flow rates of 0.12–0.16 ml/min are regarded by some to be the critical range separating individuals with salivary gland hypofunction from those with normal gland function [28]; for stimulated whole saliva this would be around 0.5 ml/min.

The most remarkable finding of all studies is the enormous variability of flow rates for both basal (unstimulated) and stimulated secretions. Throughout these vast ranges of flow rate, individuals are generally free of subjective complaints and objective signs of salivary glands dysfunction (Table 1.4; see also Sect. 1.4.4). Thus it is clear that a wide range of saliva production can allow normal oral function. Because of this heterogeneity, it is difficult to assess the status of a patient's salivary gland function from a single measurement of flow rate. In the absence of signs or symptoms, it is difficult to say whether or not this patient has a salivary gland disorder.

The stimulated whole salivary flow rate seems to be more influenced by factors such as medication than by aging [31].

It is evident that caution should be exercised in comparing a single flow rate with a population standard. It is much more likely that changes in salivary flow over time are a reliable indicator of a patient's oral health. If clinicians were to routinely assess saliva production in all of their patients, they would be able to establish a patient's normal flow rate and thus to recognize declining flow. This would allow early intervention to prevent or limit deleterious consequences of salivary gland dysfunction.

Table 1.3. Flow rates of saliva (ml/min) [7]

	Unstimulated		Stimulated	
	Mean	Range	Mean	Range
Whole saliva	0.32	0.1–0.5	1.7[a]	1.1–3.0
Parotid saliva (each gland)	0.04	0.01–0.07	1.5[b]	0.7–2.3
Submandibular/sublingual side	0.10	0.02–0.20	0.8[b]	0.4–1.3

[a] Masticatory stimulus.
[b] Gustatory stimulus (acid).

Table 1.4. Symptoms associated with salivary gland hypofunction [35]

Oral symptoms associated with salivary gland hypofunction
    Principal symptoms
        Dry mouth (xerostomia)
        Often thirsty
        Difficulty with swallowing (dysphagia)
        Difficulty with speaking (dysphonia)
        Difficulty with eating dry foods
        Need to frequently sip water while eating
        Difficulty with wearing dentures
        Often do things to keep mouth moist
    Other symptoms
        Burning, tingling sensations, especially on the tongue
        Abnormal taste sensations (dysgeusia)
        Keep fluids at bedside at night
        Fissures and sores at corners of lips
Nonoral symptoms associated with xerostomia and salivary gland hypofunction
    Dry throat
    Eyes: blurred vision; burning, itching sensations; sandy, gritty feeling in eyes;
        regular use of eye drops
    Vagina: dryness, itching, burning; history of recurrent vaginitis
    Dry skin
    Often feel constipated
    Nasal dryness

In dealing with patients with unknown normal flow rates, the clinician must utilize whatever information is available that might indicate the status of the patient's salivary function. Indicators of abnormality include certain signs and symptoms of oral desiccation as well as the salivary flow rates.

1.3.4 Measurement of Salivary Gland Function by Scintigraphy

Salivary scintigraphy measures the uptake, concentration, and secretion by the salivary glands of an intravenously injected radionuclide, e.g., ^{99m}Tc-pertechnetate. It is an excellent way to compare the functional activity of the major glands and is usually performed in a hospital setting.

1.4 Hyposalivation and Xerostomia

1.4.1 Definition and Criteria

Hyposalivation refers to a measurable decrease in function of one or more salivary glands, as reflected in the flow rate. In daily practice it is difficult for the clinician to decide whether a patient has salivary gland hypofunction; hence additional salivary gland evaluation is required, including sialometry. Navazesh et al. [28] identified a set of clinical measures that, together, successfully predicts the presence or absence of salivary gland hypofunction:

1. Dryness of lips
2. Dryness of buccal mucosa
3. Absence of saliva produced by gland palpation
4. High total decayed/missing filled teeth (DMFT) score

The term xerostomia refers to the patient's (subjective) feeling of oral dryness. In a study of 71 patients complaining of dry mouth, decreased salivary rate of flow was found in 56 [34]. In experiments designed to reduce saliva production in healthy volunteers by means of an anticholinergic drug, it was observed that the symptom of dry mouth appeared when flow was reduced to about 50% of the pre-experimental flow rate [5]. A subject with a high resting flow rate of 0.6 ml/min complained of oral dryness when the flow rate fell to a level of 0.3 ml/min; a person with a low resting flow rate of 0.2 ml/min noted that his mouth felt dry when the flow fell to 0.1 ml/min. The pH and the compostion of the saliva, particularly with regard to the potassium content, probably also play a role in the patient's experience of xerostomia [14].

There are a large number of oral and nonoral symptoms that may be associated with xerostomia and salivary gland hypofunction (Table 1.4). Many of these symptoms may also be present in patients without xerostomia, but they are much more common in those with it. Xerostomic patients complain, on average, of 3.2 symptoms each, and nonxerostomic patients of 0.8 symptoms each. With rare exceptions, e.g., in mouthbreathers and patients given therapeutic irradiation, these symptoms reflect the presence of generalized desiccation. The *oral* symptoms are due to a decrease in the functioning of the salivary glands. The *nonoral* symptoms are due to the diminution of exocrine secretion in other parts of the body. However, whether the presenting symptom is oral, e.g., xerostomia, or nonoral, e.g., vaginal dryness, the underlying cause is most likely generalized exocrine hypofunction.

A useful test for true dryness of the oral mucosa is to place a dental mirror or gloved finger against the buccal mucosa; this should lift off easily when saliva is present in normal amounts [18]. Others have used a specially designed device to register oral mucosal surface sliding friction [13, 29]. Chronic hyposalivation is a prerequisite for the usefulness of this method.

As has already been mentioned, oral dryness is sensed when the flow of saliva is decreased to about half of the subject's normal flow rate. In order for the resting flow of saliva to fall to such a level, more than one gland must be affected. The loss of activity of a single gland, seen in cases of salivary gland tumors and sialoliths, does not result in oral dryness.

1.4.2 Prevalence

The prevalence of a subjective feeling of dry mouth has been studied in various populations [8]. In Finland, 46% of an elderly population consisting of 243 women and 98 men, ranging in age from 75 to 85 years, had noticed subjective symptoms of dry mouth; 12% reported continuous oral dryness [26]. In this study, continuous dry mouth was clearly associated with the female gender, with mouth-breathing, and with the use of systemic medications.

In an American study involving 600 subjects, ranging in age from 65 to over 90 years (mean, 78 years), 39% reported having occasional mouth dryness [11]. The sex distribution was not described. Gilbert et al. [11] felt a need for investigators to standardize questions designed to measure the prevalence of xerostomia. In yet another study it was shown that the complaint of oral dryness is certainly not limited to the elderly [37].

1.4.3 Etiology

Xerostomia is usually the result of multiglandular salivary hypofunction; it is induced by systemic diseases and conditions, therapeu-

Table 1.5. The principal causes of salivary gland hypofunction and xerostomia [35]

Cause	Examples and comments
Systemic diseases	
Rheumatoid conditions	Collagen/vascular, connective tissue diseases, e.g., Sjögren's syndrome
Dysfunction of the immune system	AIDS
Hormonal disorders	Diabetes mellitus
Neurological disorders	Parkinson's disease
Dehyration	
Therapeutic irradiation	External beam, whole-body, ^{131}I
Drugs/medications	
Psychogenic disorders	Depression
Ageing	Contributory factor; probably does not induce xerostomia per se
Decreased mastication	

AIDS, acquired immunodeficiency syndrome.

tic irradiation of the head and neck, drugs, or psychogenic disorders (Table 1.5) [18, 35, 37, 38, 46].

1.4.3.1 Systemic Diseases

Xerostomia and salivary gland hypofunction are intimately associated with a number of systemic diseases and conditions. Some of these diseases and conditions cause progressive destruction of the gland parenchyma, which in most cases is irreversible. Others may have vascular or neural effects which are transient and reversible. Included among the diseases are rheumatoid conditions (sometimes referred to as collagen–vascular, connective tissue, or autoimmune disorders), certain common diseases, e.g., diabetes mellitus (DM), certain neurological conditions, and dehydration.

The are two types of evidence for DM. Some studies have found a greater incidence of DM in xerostomic subjects than in non-xerostomic controls. Other studies, which were conducted on diabetic patients who were otherwise disease free and were taking no drugs except insulin, reported a far greater prevalence of xerostomia than in matched nondiabetic controls. Nevertheless, not all studies support the importance of DM with regard to salivary gland hypofunction [40].

The possible role of hypertension is not clear. In a small series of patients, no significant differences were found in stimulated parotid flow rates between normotensive and uncontrolled hypertensive subjects [41, 42]. However, the medicated, controlled hypertensive subjects had a significant reduction of stimulated parotid salivary flow rates compared to both the normotensive and hypertensive groups.

The prototype of the rheumatoid conditions is Sjögren's syndrome (SS). The primary form of this syndrome is characterized by salivary and lacrimal gland involvement, usually presenting as dry mouth and dry eyes. The secondary form involves at least one of these organs and, in addition, a collagen disorder, most commonly rheumatoid arthritis. Systemic lupus erythematosus, scleroderma, and primary biliary cirrhosis may also be associated with secondary SS. In the early stages of SS, there may be little change in the flow rate of saliva. As the disease advances, there is a progressive decrease in flow. This progression is due to the gradual destruction of the gland parenchyma by a lymphoreticular cell infiltration, irreversible acinar cell degeneration, and atrophy (see Chap. 3).

Rare cases of xerostomia are due to an immune-mediated response in graft versus host disease (GVHD), the xerostomia being the result of an interaction between a bone marrow transplant and salivary gland tissue. The salivary gland response is characterized by lymphoplasmocytic infiltration and necrosis of epithelial cells. The salivary gland changes following bone marrow transplantation are so consistent that the development of GVHD can be assessed in a salivary gland biopsy. The decrease in salivary flow rates due to GVHD following bone marrow transplantation is as profound as that due to radiation therapy.

In a group of 78 human immunodeficiency virus (HIV)-seropositive men, 6% showed a marked reduction in parotid flow rate; low flow rate was significantly related to oral candidiasis [23].

1.4.3.2 Therapeutic Irradiation

In patients irradiated for the treatment of head and neck cancer, xerostomia, mucositis, and dysgeusia are frequently encountered.

These signs are almost always due to treatment by external beam radiation. The effects of the radiation are dose, time, and gland dependent [22]. Xerostomia and hyposalivation may be permanent in cases of bilateral exposure of the salivary glands. It should be mentioned that, even in doses above 64 Gy with bilateral radiation fields, there are large individual differences with respect to salivary flow and discomfort of dryness [10].

The secretory cells, blood supply, and the nerves may all be affected by ionizing radiation. Serous cells are more sensitive to radiation than mucous-secreting cells. Thus the secretion produced during and after radiation is reduced in amount and is thicker.

Patients often complain of oral dryness early in their treatment; dryness gets worse as the therapy proceeds. In one study there was a 50% reduction in the resting flow rate of parotid saliva 24 h after the administration of only 225 cGy. After 6 weeks of treatment (6000 cGy/fraction), the reduction was greater than 75%. In most cases, the reduction in the function of the salivary glands and the xerostomia which accompanies it are irreversible. A reduction of salivary secretion by more than 95% has been found to persist 3 years after treatment.

1.4.3.3 Drugs/Medication

Included among the xerogenic drugs are anticholinergics, anoretics, antihistamines, antidepressants, antipsychotics, antihypertensives, diuretics, and antiparkinsonism drugs (Table 1.6). At therapeutic dosages, drugs do not damage the structure of the salivary glands. Their effects are reversible, and stopping the drugs leads to a reduction in oral dryness [36].

1.4.3.4 Psychogenic Disorders

The ability of the psychological state to depress the flow of saliva has been known since Pavlov's work. Depressive effects in states of acute anxiety may be transient. Depressive effects in chronic depression are more lasting. When no organic cause of a patient's troublesome oral dryness can be found, he or she should be advised to consult a psy-

Table 1.6. Select xerogenic medications [36]

Type	Medication	Trade names
Analgesics	Meperedine HCl	Demerol
	Alprazolam	Xanax
	Diazepam	Valium
	Triazolam	Halcion
Anorexic (amphetamine)	Methaphetamine HCl	Dexosyn
Anorexic (nonamphetamine)	Phendimetrazine tartrate	Apidex, Obezine, Trimtabs
Antiacne preparation	Isotretinoin	Accutane
Antiarthritic	Piroxicam	Feldene
Anticholinergic, antispasmodic (GI)	Atropine sulfate	
	Clidinium bromide	Quarzan
	Dicyclomine	Bentyl
	Gylcopyrrolate	Robinul
	Hyoscyamine sulfate	Anaspaz
	Propantheline bromide	pro-Banthene
	Combination drugs	Donnatal
Anticholinergic, antispasmodic (urinary)	Oxybutynin chloride	Ditropan
	Combination drugs	(Cytospaz, Urised)
Antidepressant	Tricyclics	Elavil, Pamelor, Tofranil
Antidiarrheal	Diphenoxylate HCl and atropine	Lomotil
Antihistamine	Diphenhyramine HCl	Benadryl
	Brompheniramine maleate	Dimetane; Veltane
	Combination drugs	Triaminic, Historal, Dimetapp
Antihypertensive	Clonidine HCl	Catapres
	Prazosin HCl	Minipress
Antihypertensive and diuretic	Chlonidine HCl and chlorthalidone	Combipres
	Naldolol and bendroflumethazide	Corzide
	Propanolol HCl and hydrochlorothiazide	Inderdide
Antiparkinsonism	Biperiden HCl and biperiden lactate	Akineton
	Benzatropine mesylate	Cogentin
Antipsychotic	Lithium carbonate	Lithobid
	Thioridazine	Mellaril
	Trifluoperazine	Stelazine

Table 1.6. *Continued*

Type	Medication	Trade names
Diuretics	Chlorthiazide	Diuril
	Hydrochlorhiazide	Esidrex, HydroDIURIL
	Triamterene and hydrochlorothiazide	Dyazide
Psychotherapeutic agents	Alprazolam	Xanax
	Diazepam	Valium
	Triazolam	Halcion

GI, gastrointestinal.

chologist or psychiatrist to explore possible psychogenic factors. Although psychological states can induce oral dryness, little is known about their methods of action. Depression is frequently treated with tricyclic antidepressants, which tend to aggravate the degree of oral dryness.

1.4.3.5 Ageing and Decreased Mastication

Age and decreased mastication may contribute to the feeling of oral dryness. With the possible exception of postmenopausal women, ageing per se does not seem to induce a decrease in the flow rate of whole or parotid saliva [31].

Animal and limited human studies have shown that decreased mastication (liquid diet; soft foods) leads to salivary gland atrophy and a decrease in the flow of saliva. However, the glands are not destroyed, and stimulation, e.g., by mastication, induces normal or near-normal flow rates. The important point with regard to edentia is whether or not the subject masticates his or her food. Therefore, edentia per se does not have a deleterious effect on stimulated parotid salivary flow rates [39].

1.4.4 Clinical Signs Associated with Xerostomia and Salivary Gland Hypofunction

The clinical signs associated with xerostomia and salivary gland hypofunction are as follows:

- Dryness of lining oral tissues
- Loss of glistening of the oral mucosa
- Dryness of the oral mucous membranes
- Oral mucosa appears thin and pale
- Tongue blade or mirror or a gloved finger may adhere to the soft tissues
- Fissuring and lobulation of the dorsum of the tongue and, occasionally, the lips (Fig. 1.2)
- Angular cheilitis
- Candidiasis, especially on the tongue and palate
- Increase in dental caries, located at sites generally not susceptible to decay
- Thicker, more stringy whole saliva
- Difficulty in "milking" saliva from the ducts of the major salivary glands
- Swelling of the salivary glands

Patients with xerostomia may also demonstrate a wide variety of nonoral clinical signs. Eye changes include xerophthalmia, keratoconjunctivitis, decreased lacrimation, and the accumulation of viscous secretions in the conjunctival sac. Involvement of the exocrine glands may lead to pharyngitis and laryngitis, persistent hoarseness, a dry cough, and difficulty with speech. Nasal dryness may induce the

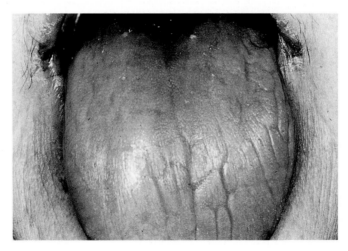

Fig. 1.2. Dryness of the dorsal surface of the tongue and angular cheilitis

formation of crusts, epistaxis, and loss of olfactory acuity. A decrease in the production of saliva as well as in secretions from the gastrointestinal tract may lead to reflux esophagitis, dyspepsia, and constipation.

1.4.5 Treatment of Xerostomia and Hyposalivation

Before any type of treatment or investigation is instituted, the patient should be well informed about the often contradictory subjective feeling of dryness and yet normal function of the salivary glands.

Therapies designed to stimulate secretion, whether local or systemic, have the great advantage of providing the benefits of natural saliva. Since salivary glands are highly responsive to stimulation of taste, of masticatory muscles, and of the sensory nerves of the mucosa and periodontium, local stimulation should be attempted first.

1.4.5.1 Local Stimulation

Chewing gum, mints, or inert substances such as paraffin or sucking a solid object such as a plum stone stimulates salivation. Most commonly, the substances (sialogogues) recommended are chewing gum, mints, and lozenges and rinses containing citric acid [1]. However, the effects are short-lived and frequent applications are required. In some patients, substances such as citric acid may irritate the mucosa, particularly if it is already sensitive due to dryness. If used often, it may contribute to tooth demineralization. Patients must be cautioned to avoid sugar-containing sialogogues, as these will exacerbate the risk of increased caries.

1.4.5.2 Systemic Stimulation

There has been increasing interest in systemic pharmacologic stimulants of salivary function. In particularly, pilocarpine hydrochloride has been examined in greater detail [9]. It is a parasympatheticomimetic drug which functions primarily as a muscarinic/cholinergic agonist with mild β-adrenergic stimulatory properties.

Pilocarpine hydrochloride is a stimulant of exocrine secretion. It has been shown to increase salivary output in healthy volunteers and to be effective in relieving oral dryness in patients with salivary gland hypofunction. However, pilocarpine will only be effective if there is a sufficient amount of remaining functional salivary tissue. Insufficient functional tissue may be present in the late stages of SS or following head and neck radiotherapy. Additionally, possible interactions with other medications or potential adverse cardiovascular and pulmonary effects limit the patient population appropriate for pilocarpine treatment. Therefore, pilocarpine hydrochloride should be used under the care of a specialist and following medical assessment.

Tablets containing 2.5–5 mg pilocarpine administered with water three times a day at meal times for a 12-week period, starting the day of or the day before radiotherapy commences, improve saliva production and relieve symptoms of xerostomia after irradiation for cancer of the head and neck. Minor side effects occur, predominantly limited to sweating [43]. Favorable results have also been published for the use of pilocarpine in irradiated patients in whom radiotherapy had been completed at least 3 months before treatment was commenced [17, 20].

Yohimbine treatment, an indole alkaloid selective antagonist for α_2-adrenoceptors, at a dosage of 4 mg three times daily for 3 weeks, may have a potential therapeutic use in treatment of dry mouth caused by tricyclic antidepressant drugs [2, 32].

1.4.5.3 Symptomatic Therapies

In the absence of natural salivation, it is essential to try to protect the oral hard and soft tissues by salivary substitution. Saliva substitutes, also called artificial salivas, are frequently employed in patients complaining of dry mouth. A number of studies have examined subjective responses to carboxymethylcellulose-based preparations or have compared these with agents containing animal mucins [30]. Although many studies suggest that saliva substitutes are useful in the management of xerostomia, clinical experience has shown that these products are often not well accepted by patients. Most patients do not continue their regular use, relying instead on water or other fluids to relieve their symptoms. Furthermore, artifical salivas fail to provide the broad spectrum of antimicrobial and other protective functions of natural saliva.

Frequent sips of water or other fluids for the relief of oral dryness are often as effective as saliva substitutes. Patients should be advised to carry fluids with them at all times. (The water bottles used by cyclists or plastic glasses with snap-on lids are convenient). This simple suggestion often brings substantial relief at minimal cost, improves mucosal hydration, and eases swallowing and speaking. Individuals should be cautioned to avoid fluids containing sugar, as these may increase the risk of caries.

1.4.5.4 Acupuncture

In a Swedish study of 21 patients with severe xerostomia, the use of acupuncture resulted in improved salivary flow rates [4]. The improved salivary values persisted during the observation year, whereas the patients who received placebo acupuncture showed some improvement of salivary flow rates only during the actual treatment.

1.5 Hypersalivation

Occasionally, patients complain of hypersalivation, i.e., excessive saliva production (sialorrhea, ptyalism). Individuals reporting such complaints usually do not demonstrate salivary flow rates which exceed the normal range. Rather, such complaints reflect problems in oral motor coordination, including reduced muscle tone around the mouth and a reduced ability to swallow. For instance, sialorrhea after extensive surgery for oral or oropharyngeal disorders seems to be the result of impaired swallowing function rather than excessive production of saliva.

In some patients, the excessive saliva is episodic in nature, with paroxysms of secretion occurring once or twice a week and lasting a few minutes [21]. A fairly common cause of episodic hypersalivation is gastroesophageal reflux (GER), which is frequently associated with pregnancy and hiatal hernia [24].

Sialorrhea can be the result of stomatitis, psychological factors, and the use of some drugs, e.g., benzodiazepines and captopril [3].

There is no evidence that relates hypersalivation to personality, at least not in volunteers selected from a nonmedicated, nonpsychiatric population [25]. Increased salivation is a recognized problem in patients who have diabetic autonomic neuropathy, Parkinson's disease, or cerebral palsy [18] (Fig. 1.3). In some patients, however, no distinct cause can be detected.

As with xerostomia, the patient's experience of suffering from excessive saliva production cannot and should not be denied by the clinician, even if there is an apparently normal wetting of the oral mucosa. Explaining the mechanisms of saliva production and the complexity of salivary gland function to the patient may produce benefits.

It is quite difficult to decrease the production of saliva. The use of drugs, such as atropine, is rather unattractive because of adverse side effects. Hypersalivation induced by clozapine, a broad-spectrum antipsychotic, may be successfully treated by application of a clonidine patch (0.1 mg once a week) [12]. Submandibular duct diversion is a fairly common procedure for patients with refractory sialorrhea, e.g., patients suffering from cerebral palsy. The procedure reroutes Wharton's ducts from the floor of the mouth to the base of the tongue with or without extirpation of both sublingual glands [15]. The results of this procedure are satisfactory [16]. A further,

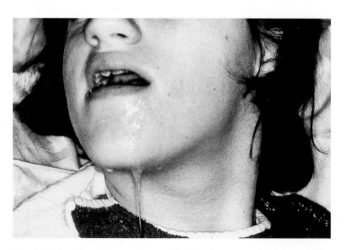

Fig. 1.3. Drooling in a patient suffering from cerebral palsy. (From [16] with permission)

more complicated procedure consists of rerouting of the Stensen's duct and bilateral removal of the submandibular salivary glands, as described by Wilkie and Brody [44] and reported by various authors [6, 33].

References

1. Aagaard A, Godiksen S, Teglers PT, et al. Comparison between new saliva stimulants in patients with dry mouth: a placebo-controlled double-blind crossover study. J Oral Pathol Med 1992; 21: 376–380.
2. Bagheri H, Schmitt L, Berlan M, et al. Effect of 3 weeks treatment with yohimbine on salivary secretion in healthy volunteers and in depressed patients treated with tricyclic antidepressant. Br J Clin Pharmacol 1992; 34: 555–558.
3. Biron P. Intermittent cough, sulfur-tasting sputum, and hypersalivation associated with captopril. Arch Intern Med 1988; 148: 245–246.
4. Blom M, Dawidson I, Angmar-Mansson B. The effect of acupuncture on salivary flow rates in patients with xerostomia. Oral Surg Oral Med Oral Pathol 1992; 73: 293–298.
5. Dawes C. Physiological factors affecting salivary flow rate, oral sugar clearance and the sensation of dry mouth in man. J Dent Res 1987; 66: 648–653.
6. Dundas DF, Peterson RA. Surgical treatment of drooling by bilateral parotid duct ligation and submandibular gland resection. Plastic and Reconstructive Surg 1979; 64: 47–51.
7. Edgar WM. Saliva: its secretion, composition and functions. Br Dent J 1992; 172: 305–312.
8. Fox PC, Ven van der PF, Sonies BC, et al. Xerostomia: evaluation of a symptom with increasing significance. JADA 1985; 110: 519–525.
9. Fox PC, Ven van der PF, Baum BJ, et al. Pilocarpine for the treatment of xerostomia associated with salivary gland dysfunction. Oral Surg Oral Med Oral Pathol 1986; 61: 243–248.
10. Franzén L, Funegård U, Ericson T, et al. Parotid gland function during and following radiotherapy of malignancies in the head and neck. A consecutive study of salivary flow and patient discomfort. Eur J Cancer 1992; 28: 457–462.
11. Gilbert GH, Heft MW, Duncan RP. Mouth dryness as reported by older Floridians. Community Dent Oral Epidemiol 1993; 21: 390–397.
12. Grabowski J. Clonidine treatment of clozapine-induced hypersalivation. J Clin Psychopharmacol 1992; 12: 69–70.
13. Henricsson V, Svensson A, Olsson H, et al. Evaluation of a new device for measuring oral mucosal surface friction. Scand J Dent Res 1990; 98: 529–536.
14. Hornstein OP. Chronische Mundtrockenheit – Klinische und Therapeutische Probleme. Dtsch Z Mund-Kiefer-Gesichts-Chir 1981; 4: 14–20.
15. Hotaling AJ, Madgy DN, Kuhns LR, et al. Postoperative Technetium scanning in patients with submandibular duct diversion. Arch Otolaryngol Head Neck Surg 1992; 118: 1331–1333.

16. Jaquinet AR, Richter M, Laurent F, et al. Traitement chirurgical de l'incontinence salivaire chez l'infirme moteur cérébral. Rev Stomatol Chir maxillofac 1993; 94: 366–370.

17. Johnson JT, Ferretti GA, Nethery WJ, et al. Oral pilocarpine for post-irradiation xerostomia in patients with head and neck cancer. N Engl J Med 1993; 329: 390–395.

18. Lamey P-J, Lewis MAO. Oral medicine in practice: salivary gland disease. Br Dent J 1990; 168: 237–243.

19. Laudenbach P, Huynh D. Pour une débitmétrie salivaire pratique, Une technique pondérale. Rev Stomatol Chir maxillofac 1994; 95: 130–133.

20. LeVeque FG, Montgomery M, Potter D, et al. A multicenter, randomized, double-blind, placebo-controlled, dose-titration study of oral pilocarpine for treatment of radiation-induced xerostomia in head and neck cancer patients. J Clin Oncol 1993; 11: 1124–1131.

21. Lieblich S. Episodic supersalivation (idiopathic paroxysmal sialorrhea): Description of a new clinical syndrome. Oral Surg Oral Med Oral Pathol 1989; 68: 159–161.

22. Liu RP, Fleming TJ, Toth BB, et al. Salivary flow rates in patients with head and neck cancer 0.5 to 25 years after radiotherapy. Oral Surg Oral Med Oral Pathol 1990; 70: 724–729.

23. Mandel ID, Barr CE, Turgeon L. Longitudinal study of parotid saliva in HIV-1 infection. J Oral Pathol Med 1992; 21: 209–213.

24. Mandel L, Tamari K. Sialorrhea and gastroesophageal reflux. JADA 1995; 126: 1537–1541.

25. Millar K, Greddes DAM, Hammersley RH, et al. Is salivary flow related to personality? Br Dent J 1993; 175: 13–19.

26. Närhi TO. Prevalence of subjective feelings of dry mouth in the elderly. J Dent Res 1994; 73: 20–25.

27. Navazesh M, Christensen C. A comparison of whole mouth resting and stimulated salivary measurement procedures. J Dent Res 1982; 61: 1158–1162.

28. Navazesh M, Christensen C, Brightman V. Clinical criteria for the diagnosis of salivary gland hypofunction. J Dent Res 1992; 71(7): 1363–1369.

29. Nederfors T, Henricsson V, Dahlöf C, et al. Oral mucosal friction and subjective perception of dry mouth in relation to salivary secretion. Scand J Dent Res 1993; 101: 44–48.

30. Olsson H, Axéll T. Objective and subjective efficacy of saliva substitutes containing mucin and carboxymethylcellulax. Scand J Dent Res 1991; 99: 316–319.

31. Persson RE, Izutsu KT, Truelove EL, et al. Differences in salivary flow rates in elderly subjects using xerostomatic medications. Oral Surg Oral Med Oral Pathol 1991; 72: 42–46.

32. Rispail Y, Schmitt L, Berlan M, et al. Yohimbine increases salivary secretion in depressed patients treated with tricyclic antidepressants. Eur J Clin Pharmacol 1990; 39: 425–426.

33. Rosen A, Kominsar A, Ophir D, et al. Experience with the Wilkie procedure for sialorrhea. Ann Otol Rhinol Laryngol 1990; 99: 730–732.

34. Spielman A, Ben-Aryeh H, Gutman D et al. Xerostomia – Diagnosis and treatment. Oral Surg Oral Med Oral Pathol 1981; 51: 144–147.

35. Sreebny LM (ed). Saliva: its role in health and disease. Int Dent J 1992; 42 (suppl. 2): 291–304.

36. Sreebny LM, Schwartz SS. Reference guide to drugs and dry mouth. Gerodontol 1986; 5: 75–99.

37. Sreebny LM, Valdini A. Xerostomia. Part I: Relationship to other oral symptoms and salivary gland hypofunction. Oral Surg Oral Med Oral Pathol 1988; 66: 451–458.

38. Sreebny LM, Valdini A. Xerostomia. Part II: Relationship to nonoral symptoms, drugs, and diseases. Oral Surg Oral Med Oral Pathol 1989; 68: 419–427.

39. Streckfus CF, Brown LJ, Ship JA, et al. Stimulated parotid gland flow rates in healthy, elderly dentulous and edentulous individuals. J Prosthet Dent 1993; 70: 496–499.

40. Streckfus CF, Marcus S, Welsh S, et al. Parotid function and composition of parotid saliva among elderly edentulous African-American diabetics. J Oral Pathol Med 1994; 23: 277–279.

41. Streckfus CF, Wu AJ, Ship JA, et al. Stimulated parotid salivary flow rates in normotensive, hypertensive, and hydrochlorothiazide-medicated African-Americans. J Oral Pathol Med 1994; 23: 280–283.

42. Streckfus CF, Wu AJ, Ship JA, et al. Comparison of stimulated parotid salivary gland flow rates in normotensive and hypertensive persons. Oral Surg Oral Med Oral Pathol 1994; 77: 615–619.

43. Valdez IH, Wolff A, Atkinson JC, et al. Use of pilocarpine during head and neck radiation therapy to reduce xerostomia and salivary dysfunction. Cancer 1993; 71: 1848–1851. A.

44. Wilkie TF, Brody GS. The surgical treatment of drooling. A ten-year review. Plast Recontr Surg 1977; 59: 791–798.

45. Wolff A, Fox PC, Ship JA, et al. Oral mucosal status and major salivary gland function. Oral Surg Oral Med Oral Pathol 1990; 70: 49–54.

46. Wu AJ, Ship JA. A characterization of major salivary gland flow rates in the presence of medications and systemic diseases. Oral Surg Oral Med Oral Pathol 1993; 76: 301–306.

2 Inflammatory Diseases

2.1 Introduction

Inflammation of the acino-parenchymal structures of the salivary glands is called *sialadenitis* and mainly affects the parotid and submandibular glands. Sialadenitis of the intraoral glands is rare, as is sialadenitis of the sublingual gland.

Inflammatory changes in the ducts of the salivary glands are known as *sialodochitis*.

Sialadenitis can be of an acute, a subacute, or a chronic nature and can be of bacterial or viral origin. Bacterial sialadenitis is usually subclassified according to the age of the patient, the affected gland, and the clinical course (Table 2.1). Sialadenitis can also result from allergic reactions, autoimmune reactions, reaction to irradiation of the salivary glands, or from certain drugs, such as ritodrine hydrochloride [18].

2.2 Sialadenitis of the Parotid Gland

2.2.1 Acute (Suppurative) Parotitis

Acute (suppurative) parotitis, sometimes representing an exacerbation of a chronic disease, is an ascending bacterial sialadenitis characterized by a preauricular swelling that suddenly appears, either unilaterally or bilaterally.

Primary acute parotitis has been mainly reported in elderly patients suffering from dehydration, malnutrition, liver cirrhosis, or diabetes mellitus. Acute parotitis has only occasionally been observed in premature infants [11].

Table 2.1. Classification of bacterial sialadenitis

Gland	Type of inflammation
Parotid gland	Acute (suppurative) parotitis Chronic parotitis Juvenile recurrent parotitis Adult recurrent parotitis
Submandibular gland	Chronic sialadenitis
Sublingual gland	Rarely inflamed
Intraoral salivary gland	Chronic sialadenitis, e.g., glandular cheilitis Subacute necrotizing sialadenitis

The patient experiences a fairly intense radiating pain in the affected side of the face. General malaise and fever are common. Some patients complain of limited movement of the mandible and difficulties in swallowing. In some cases disturbances of the facial nerve may be noticed.

Intraorally, an inflamed parotid papilla on the affected side can be observed. The salivary secretion is reduced and may consist of a purulent discharge.

Because of the often painful swelling, the use of sialography is discouraged.

Scintigraphic examination may show an increased intensity of the involved parotid gland. In cases involving abscess formation, an area of reduced activity may be observed. This is better seen with ultrasonographic examination.

Several microorganisms may be involved, such as the facultative anaerobic *Staphylococcus aureus* and *Streptococcus viridans*. Strict anaerobes such as *Fusobacterium nucleatum* and *Peptostreptococcus anaerobius* may also play a role [15].

Treatment consists of elimination of the cause such as a mucous plug, if it is identifiable [13]. In cases involving abcess formation, incision and drainage are indicated. Administration of a semisynthetic penicillin such as dicloxacillin is only indicated in cases of general malaise and fever.

2.2.2 Chronic Recurrent Parotitis

Chronic (adult) parotitis can follow a subclinical course. As with acute parotitis, the infection usually occurs via the excretory duct. Inflammation of the oral mucosa and a reduced salivary flow may lead to an ascending or retrograde infection in the major salivary glands. Occasionally, parotid infections are superimposed on underlying Sjögren's disease, sialadenosis, neoplasms, or the rare Darier's disease [1]. It has been suggested that adult patients with chronic parotitis, but without a history of parotid gland swelling in childhood, should be provisionally diagnosed as having subclinical Sjögren's syndrome [25].

Chronic inflammation results primarily in destruction of the serous acini. This causes a reduction in salivary production, which further facilitates extension of the infection.

A combination of a congenital malformation of portions of the salivary ducts and infections ascending from the mouth following dehydration in children are contributory to the pathogenesis of *juvenile recurrent parotitis* [7]. It seems unlikely that juvenile recurrent parotitis is an allergic condition of immature immune response, of mumps, or of sensitivity to upper respiratory tract infections. Familial and racial factors do not seem to play a role either [7]. Boys are more often affected than girls.

2.2.2.1 Clinical Aspects

Although the inflammation may occur bilaterally, the symptoms of a painful swelling are often unilateral. This is true both in chronic recurrent parotitis and in juvenile recurrent parotitis. In case involving a swelling in the parotid gland area, not only inflammatory salivary gland diseases but also salivary gland neoplasms should be considered, as well as sialadenosis and lymphadenopathies. Such lymphadenopathy may be caused by a variety of diseases, e.g., cat-scratch disease, toxoplasmosis, and primary or secondary neoplasms. Chronic sialadenitis may also be associated with salivary gland neoplasms [4].

Intraorally, an inflamed parotid papilla may be observed. The saliva may be somewhat watery with white flakes (snow storm).

Purulent discharge is rare and may be associated with diabetes mellitus.

Because the remaining salivary glands function normally, patients with chronic recurrent parotitis do not complain of xerostomia.

2.2.2.2 Bacteriological Findings

As in acute parotitis, microbiological culturing of the saliva is recommended. *Streptococcus viridans* and sometimes also pneumococci and staphylococci are often present. Involvement of specific microorganisms, such as *Myobacterium tuberculosis* [16, 20, 27] and actinomycosis [9], is quite rare. Intra- and periglandular lymph nodes are involved in such cases, but involvement of the parenchymal tissue is rare.

2.2.2.3 Sialographic Findings

Sialography, which involves the retrograde injection of a radiopaque dye into the main excretory duct, is the most important tool in establishing a diagnosis of chronic parotitis. In the parotid gland, more than 90% dilatation of ducts and less than 10% ectasias are seen, while in the submandibular gland only dilatation of ducts is observed. In addition to plain radiographs, computed tomography (CT) sialography may provide additional and more detailed information.

In some patients, widening of the major excretory ducts is observed (sialodochitis), occasionally with a colon-like ("sausage-string") structure (Fig. 2.1). In the initial stage of the disease, in which only the acini are involved, the sialogram may appear more or less normal. Based on morphologic changes in the sialograms, a division of four types of chronic (adult) parotitis can be made [28] (Table 2.2).

Sialectasia is a diagnostic feature of juvenile recurrent parotitis [12] (Fig. 2.2).

It has been suggested that sialectasis as observed on a sialogram actually represents extravasation of contrast material. The use of water-soluble contrast medium may therefore be considered, espe-

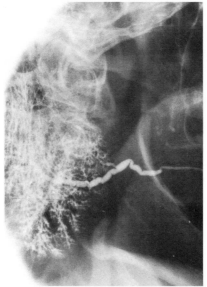

a

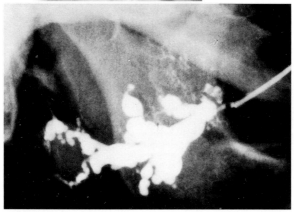

b

Fig. 2.1. a Sialogram of a mild form of chronic recurrent parotitis. Note the colon-like ("sausage-string") appearance of Stensen's duct. **b** Advanced form of chronic recurrent parotitis showing dilatation of branching ducts and disappearance of acinar structures

cially when the presence of an inflammatory disease is anticipated. Other workers, however, have not found evidence from histological material to support the hypothesis that sialectasis represents extravasation of injected fluid [7].

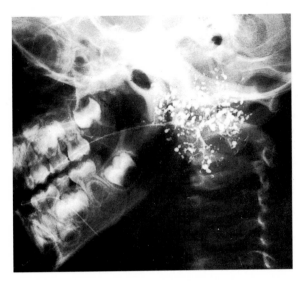

Fig. 2.2. Sialogram of juvenile recurrent parotitis. Note the extensive sialectasia

Table 2.2. Chronic (adult) obstructive parotitis [28]

Type	Features	Severity
1	Irregular dilation of main duct starting from orifice, branching ducts not involved	Relatively mild type
2	Anterior part of main duct normal, but posterior part irregularly dilated; punctate sialectasis occasionally observed	Relatively moderate severity
3	Irregular dilation of the whole main duct, often extending to branching ducts; punctate sialectasis may be observed	Relatively moderate severity
4	Severe dilatation of the whole main duct, extending into branching ducts with disappearance of acini in some cases; punctate and globular sialectasis may be present	Most severe type

2.2.2.4 Scintigraphic Findings

Scintigraphy is considered to be a useful diagnostic aid in chronic recurrent parotitis, especially in patients in whom sialography cannot be performed [23, 24].

Nuclide uptake function is increased in the mild type of chronic parotitis, while the excretory function is normal [28]. In the moderately diseased parotid gland, uptake is almost normal and excretion is obstructed or retarded. In severe types, both uptake and excretion are obstructed.

2.2.2.5 Ultrasound Examination

Ultrasound examination is not very useful in detecting chronic inflammation.

2.2.2.6 Laboratory Findings

Laboratory findings, such as hemoglobin level, leukocyte and differential counts, and erythrocyte sedimentation rate are usually normal.

2.2.2.7 Histological Aspects

In chronic parotitis, the parenchymal structures may be largely replaced by fibrosis and fat, with only some intralobular ducts remaining. The ducts are often dilated and surrounded by a dense lymphocytic infiltrate. In a study of 23 patients with chronic parotitis, the extent of the histopathologic changes largely paralleled the severity of the sialographic changes [22].

In juvenile recurrent parotitis, enlarged vacuolated acini, dilatation of the intralobular ducts, and a slight infiltration of inflammatory cells can be observed [22].

2.2.2.8 Treatment

In general, patients with chronic parotitis should be instructed to carefully massage the involved gland in a dorsoventral direction, at least five times a day, and to eat sour foods to stimulate parotid secretion. Furthermore, attention should be given to proper oral hygiene in order to reduce the chance of retrograde infection.

Although chronic parotitis in adult patients may cause severe complaints, there is rarely an indication for parotidectomy. The main reason for a nonsurgical approach is the difficulty of identifying the numerous branches of the facial nerve in the inflamed parotid gland. Some authors, however, prefer to use surgical management early rather than to wait for the formation of fistulas or abscesses [2]. Total parotidectomy with facial nerve dissection is preferred to superficial lobe parotidectomy.

Injection of 1% methylviolet into the excretory duct of the parotid gland has been used in severe cases of chronic parotitis not amenable to treatment with conservative methods. If used properly, one or two injections are reported to be sufficient in chronic parotitis; this method should not be used in juvenile recurrent parotitis [28]. Repeated injections, e.g., once per month for 6 months, of 2 ml dexamethasone in the main duct may relieve the complaints to some extent, but the effectiveness of such a regimen has not been well established.

Chronic juvenile recurrent parotitis usually regresses spontaneously at puberty. The sialographic picture may improve in time [8]. Only where extensive widening or obstruction of the excretory ducts occurs may chronic inflammation persist after puberty. Some authors have suggested calling this "recurrent parotitis in adults" (RPA) and distinguish this condition from chronic parotitis [22].

2.2.3 Epidemic Parotitis ("Mumps")

Epidemic parotitis ("mumps") is a contagious disease that is caused by a paramyxovirus. Apart from the major salivary glands, the testes, meninges, pancreas, heart, and mammary glands may become involved. It has been shown that in 30%–40% of infected patients no clinical symptoms have been noticed. In some parts of the world, infants are routinely vaccinated with a measles/mumps/rubella vaccine [5, 17].

Mumps is often preceded by a viral infection in the oral cavity or the nose, leading to viremia and hematogenous infection of the salivary glands. The "mumps" virus is transmitted by droplet infections carried in the saliva. The incubation period is approximately 3 weeks.

Mumps is predominantly a childhood disease and is more common in boys than in girls. Characteristically, it is a rather painful, nonsuppurative swelling of one or both parotid glands (Fig. 2.3). Often only one parotid gland is swollen for a few days, followed by swelling of the contralateral gland. The submandibular glands may additionally become involved. Swelling of the affected glands may persist for 1–2 weeks. The fever often associated with the swelling lasts only for a few days to 1 week.

The virus can be isolated from the saliva during the first week of the clinical manifestation of the disease. During this period, serological examination should be performed, using a complement-binding reaction. A titer of more than 1:192 indicates recent infection [3].

In approximately 20% of adult men with mumps, orchitis and/or epididymitis may occur. In only 10% of those patients is there any bilateral involvement, in 1% resulting in complete sterility. Meningoencephalitis, mastitis, nephritis, and pancreatitis are other well-known complications of the disease. However, in general the course of the disease is benign.

Apart from vaccination, no effective treatment for mumps is available. It is a self-limiting condition, which produces life-long immunity.

2.3 Sialadenitis of the Submandibular Gland

Most cases of sialadenitis of the submandibular gland are associated with or due to the formation of a calculus (sialolithiasis). Subman-

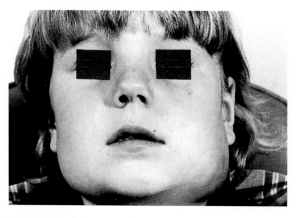

Fig. 2.3. Clinical aspect of mumps

dibular sialoadenitis has occasionally been described in patients taking iodine-containing expectorants [19]. In cases of chronic, mild inflammation, the gland is somewhat indurated and may produce a tumor-like swelling, known as Küttner tumor or inflammatory pseudotumor [10]. Symptoms are usually mild or absent. Swelling in the region of the angle of the mandible may also be caused by a neoplasm of the submandibular gland or lymphadenopathy.

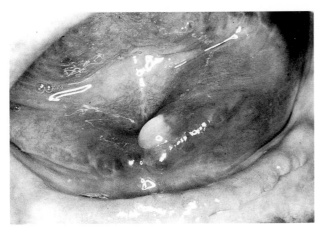

Fig. 2.4. Purulent discharge from submandibular duct orifice

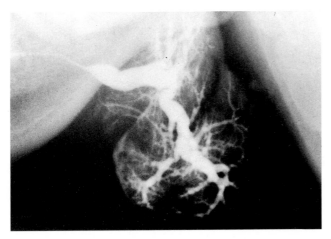

Fig. 2.5. Sialogram of chronic sialadenitis of the submandibular gland showing widening of ducts

The secretion of the gland can be somewhat diminished and may consist of a purulent discharge (Fig. 2.4).

A sialogram will show a widened Wharton's duct. In contrast to the parotid gland, no colon-like strictures of the main duct of the submandibular gland are found, whereas sialoectasis is almost never seen (Fig. 2.5). Specific inflammatory reactions in the submandibular gland rarely occur.

On histological examination, interlobular fibrosis can be seen. The lobular architecture of the parenchyme remains intact, although atrophy of the acini can be very distinct. The excretory ducts are often dilated, while the epithelial lining cells may show mucous metaplasia. There is usually a dense periductal lymphocytic infiltration.

2.4 Sialadenitis of the Sublingual Gland

Inflammation of the sublingual gland is extremely rare, possibly because of the high mucin content of its secretion and the short excretory ducts.

2.5 Sialadenitis of the Intraoral Salivary Glands

Although the intraoral salivary glands may undergo the same pathologic changes as those observed in the major glands, inflammatory changes are quite rare. They may be involved, however, in diffuse inflammatory processes of the mucosa and submucosa of the oral cavity, especially of the labial mucosa and the commissures. In the latter case, the term *glandular cheilitis* is used, also referred to as *suppurative stomatitis glandularis* [14]. Sialadenitis of palatal salivary glands may possibly be caused by tobacco use [6].

A few cases of so-called *subacute necrotizing sialadenitis* (SANS) of the palate have been reported [26]. Typically, the lesion presents as a painful unilateral, firm nodule measuring 0.3–1.0 cm in the glandular area of the hard palate (Fig. 2.6). SANS is probably not an entity on its own and should instead be regarded within the category of necrotizing sialometaplasias (see Chap. 5) [21].

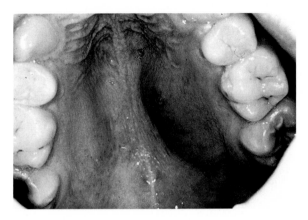

Fig. 2.6. Palatal swelling of some days duration. Biopsy revealed the presence of subacute necrotizing sialadenitis

Light microscopy examination reveals a subacute inflammatory process involving the minor salivary glands. There is loss of acinar cells. The duct cells do not show hyperplasia or metaplasia.

No treatment is necessary. Spontaneous healing occurs within 1–2 weeks.

References

1. Adams AM, Macleod RI, Munro CS. Symptomatic and asymptomatic salivary duct abnormalities in Darier's disease: a sialographic study. Dentomaxillofac Radiol 1994; 23: 25–28.
2. Arriaga MA, Myers EN. The surgical management of chronic parotitis. Laryngoscope 1990; 100: 1270–1275.
3. Batsakis JG. Tumors of the Head and Neck. Clinical and Pathological Considerations, 2nd ed. The Williams and Wilkins Company, Baltimore, 1979.
4. Batsakis JG. Granulomatous sialadenitis. Ann Otol Rhinol Laryngol 1991; 100: 166–169.
5. Druten van JAM, Boo de Th, Plantinga AD. Measles, mumps and rubella: control by vaccination. Dev Biol Stand 1986; 65: 53–63.
6. Eliasson L, Heyden G, Landahl S, et al. Effects of tobacco and diuretics on human palatal salivary glands. J Oral Pathol Med 1991; 20: 126–129.
7. Ericson S, Zetterlund B, Öhman J. Recurrent parotitis and sialectasis in childhood. Clinical, radiologic, immunologic, bacteriologic, and histologic study. Ann Otol Rhinol Laryngol 1991; 100: 527–535.

8. Geterud A, Lindvall A-M, Nylén O. Follow-up study of recurrent parotitis in children. Ann Otol Rhinol Laryngol 1988; 97: 341–346.
9. Hensher R, Bowerman J. Actinomycosis of the parotid gland. Br J Oral Maxillofac Surg 1985; 23: 128–134.
10. Inui M, Tagawa T, Mori A, et al. Inflammatory pseudotumor in the submandibular region. Clinicopathologic study and review of the literature. Oral Surg Oral Med Oral Pathol 1993; 76: 333–337.
11. Kaban LB, Mullikan JB, Murray JE. Sialadenitis in childhood. Am J Surg 1978; 135: 570–576.
12. Lamey P-J, Lewis MAO. Oral medicine in practice: salivary gland disease. Br Dent J 1990; 168: 237–243.
13. Langlais RP, Benson BW, Barnett DA. Salivary gland dysfunction: infections, sialoliths, and tumor. Ear, Nose and Throat Journal 1989; 68: 758–770.
14. Lederman DA. Suppurative stomatis glandularis. Oral Surg Oral Med Oral Pathol 1994; 78: 319–322.
15. Lewis MAO, Lamey P-J, Gibson J. Quantitative bacteriology of a case of acute parotitis. Oral Surg Oral Med Oral Pathol 1989; 68: 571–575.
16. Marrakchi R, Fathallah M, Touati S, et al. La tuberculose parotidienne. A propos de 2 cas. Rev Stomatol Chir maxillofac 1989; 90: 297–299.
17. Miller E, Goldacre M, Pugh S, et al. Risk of aseptic meningitis after measles, mumps, and rubella vaccine in UK children. Lancet 1993; 341: 979–982.
18. Minakami H, Takahashi T, Izumi A, et al. Enlargement of the salivary gland after ritodrine treatment in pregnant women. BMJ 1992; 304: 1668.
19. Soresso DJ, Mehta JB. Sialoadenitis: a rare but well-recognized complication of iodinated glycerol. Ann Otol Rhinol Laryngol 1995; 104: 162–163.
20. Taher AA. Tuberculosis of the parotid salivary gland – case report. Br J Oral Maxillofac Surg 1988; 26: 514–516.
21. Wal van der JE, Kraaijenhagen HA, Waal van der I. Subacute necrotizing sialadenitis; a new entity? Br J Oral Maxillofac Surg 1995; 33: 302–303.
22. Wang SL, Zou ZJ, Wu QG, et al. Histopathologic findings in a case of recurrent parotitis in adulthood. J Oral Maxillofac Surg 1992; 50: 1332–1333.
23. Wang SL, Zou ZJ, Wu QC, et al. Sialographic changes related to clinical and pathologic findings in chronic obstructive parotitis. Int J Oral Maxillofac Surg 1992; 21: 364–368.
24. Wang SL, Zou ZJ, Zhu J. Sequential quantitative scintigraphy of parotid glands with chronic inflammatory diseases. J Oral Maxillofac Surg 1992; 50: 456–465.
25. Wang SL, Zou ZJ, Yu SF, et al. Recurrent swelling of parotid glands and Sjögren's syndrome. Int J Oral Maxillofac Surg 1993; 22: 362–365.
26. Werning JT, Waterhouse JP, Mooney JW. Subacute necrotizing sialadenitis. Oral Surg Oral Med Oral Pathol 1990; 70: 756–759.
27. Zhen JW, Zhang QH. Tuberculosis of the parotid gland: a report of 12 cases. J Oral Maxillofac Surg 1995; 53: 849–851.
28. Zou Z, Wang S, Zhu J, et al. Chronic obstructive parotitis. Report of ninety-two cases. Oral Surg Oral Med Oral Pathol 1992; 73: 434–440.

3 Sjögren's Syndrome

3.1 Definition

Sjögren's syndrome (SS) is a chronic inflammatory disorder of salivary glands and tear glands, reflecting general involvement of exocrine tissues and leading to functional impairment. Since all exocrine glands of the body are involved, some authors prefer the use of the term inflammatory exocrinopathy.

SS usually is subclassified into two entities. The *primary type*, also called sicca syndrome, consists of xerostomia and xerophthalmia (keratoconjunctivitis sicca); in the *secondary type* there is, in addition to the features described for primary SS, evidence of a connective tissue disease such as rheumatoid arthritis or other idiopathic autoimmune diseases such as systemic lupus erythematosus, periarteritis nodosa, polymyositis, dermatomyositis, or progressive systemic sclerosis.

There is currently no international consensus about the criteria of SS. However, preliminary criteria for the classification of SS have been published by a European Study Group [50]; these criteria are listed in Table 3.1. According to these criteria, a diagnosis of primary SS should be based on at least four of the six items listed, accepting as serologic parameters only positive anti-Ro/SS-A and anti-La/SS-B antibodies. A positive response to one of the first two items (ocular and/or oral symptoms) plus a positive response to at least two of the next three items (ocular signs, histopathologic features, and salivary gland involvement) in Table 3.1 results in a diagnosis of secondary SS.

3.2 Etiology

The etiology of SS is not well understood. Several factors are thought to be of importance, e.g., hormonal disturbances, neuroendocrino-

Table 3.1. Preliminary criteria for the classification of Sjögren's syndrome (SS) [50]

Symptoms	Definition
Ocular symptoms	A positive response to at least one of the following three questions: (a) Have you had daily, persistent, troublesome dry eyes for more than 3 months? (b) Do you have a recurrent sensation of sand or gravel in the eyes? (c) Do you use tear substitutes more than three times a day?
Oral symptoms	A positive response to at least one of the following three questions: (a) Have you had a daily feeling of dry mouth for more than 3 months? (b) Have you had recurrent or persistently swollen salivary glands as an adult? (c) Do you frequently drink liquids to aid in swallowing dry foods?
Ocular signs	Objective evidence of ocular involvement, determined on the basis of a positive result on at least one of the following two tests: (a) Schirmer-1 test (5 mm or less in 5 min) (b) Rose bengal score (4 or higher, according to the Van Bijsterveld scoring system)
Histopathologic features	Focus score of 1 or more on minor salivary gland biopsy (focus defined as an agglomeration of at least 50 mononuclear cells; focus score defined as the number of foci per $4 \, mm^2$ glandular tissue)
Salivary gland involvement	Objective evidence of salivary gland involvement, determined on the basis of a positive result on at least one of the following three tests: (a) Salivary scintigraphy (b) Parotid sialography (c) Unstimulated salivary flow (1.5 ml or less in 15 min)
Autoantibodies	Presence of at least one of the following serum autoantibodies: (a) Antibodies to Ro/SS-A or La/SS-B antigens (b) Antinuclear antibodies (c) Rheumatoid factor

Exclusion criteria: preexisting lymphoma, acquired immunodeficiency syndrome (AIDS), sarcoidosis, or graft versus host disease (GVHD).

Primary SS is classified as the presence of four of the above six items, accepting as serologic parameters (see 'Autoantibodies') only positive anti-Ro/SS-A and anti-La/SS-B antibodies.

Secondary SS is classified as a positive response to the first and/or second item (ocular and/or oral symptoms), plus a positive response to at least two of the next three items (ocular signs, histopathologic features, and salivary gland involvement).

logical factors, and autoimmunity. In a study in Japan, human T lymphotropic virus-1 (HTLV-1) has been shown to play a role in the pathogenesis of SS [47]. HTLV-1 contributes to the development of various inflammatory disorders.

3.3 Epidemiology

Primary SS has a worldwide distribution and may have a frequency as high as 1:3000 [21]. SS has a strong preference for occurrence in middle-aged women. Occurrence in children and adolescents is rare [38]. Familial occurrence of the disease is also rare [32].

3.4 Clinical Aspects

3.4.1 Ocular Symptoms

Keratoconjunctivitis sicca (KCS) may cause a dry, burning, or sandy sensation in the eyes. Signs and symptoms of KCS may also be caused by diseases other than SS.

3.4.2 Oral and Perioral Symptoms

In the majority of patients with SS, xerostomia is one of the major complaints. The salivary dysfunction is due to lymphosialadeno-pathy, which includes autoimmune lymphocytic infiltration of the salivary gland parenchyme.

In 25% of patients there is a unilateral or bilateral recurrent swelling of the parotid glands, which is usually not painful to palpation (Fig. 3.1). In such glands, inflammatory changes and calculus formation may develop as a secondary phenomenon. It has been suggested that patients with adult recurrent sialadenitis of the parotid glands, but without a history of parotid gland swellings in childhood, should be provisionally diagnosed as having subclinical SS [51]. Because human immunodeficiency virus (HIV)-associated salivary gland disease can clinically resemble SS, the differential diagnosis of bilateral parotid enlargement should include HIV

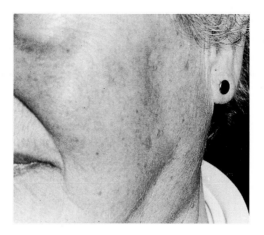

Fig. 3.1. Diffuse enlargement of parotid gland in patient suffering from Sjögren's syndrome

infection [40]. Sialadenosis, as sometimes seen in bulimia and anorexia nervosa, may also result in painless bilateral parotid enlargement.

Patients with salivary dysfunction associated with SS often complain of dysphagia [33]. Other oral manifestations include lobulation of the dorsal surface of the tongue, mucositis, dysgeusia, and angular cheilitis. Furthermore, early dental loss may reflect a silent involvement of the salivary glands and suggests that changes in saliva biochemistry occur long before xerostomia becomes clinically evident [8].

3.4.3 General Manifestations

Fatigue and general malaise are common complaints in patients with SS. In patients with secondary SS, the sicca symptoms are usually less severe than those of the accompanying autoimmune disease.

A few cases of SS associated with pulmonary hypertension have been reported [39]. Furthermore, involvement of the salivary glands has been observed in a considerable percentage of patients with autoimmune thyroiditis [52]. The spectrum of patients with a differential diagnosis of SS includes the following [20]:

1. Patients with sicca problems due to autonomic neuropathy associated with diabetes mellitus

2. Patients who have a systemic autoimmune disorder and have anti-nuclear antibodies, but who lack significant sicca symptoms or a significant focal lymphocytic infiltrate in their salivary glands
3. Patients with increased sicca symptoms associated with poorly understood dysfunction of their autonomic neural function, including stress reactions and depression
4. Patients receiving medications or nutritional supplements with anticholinergic side effects

3.5 Diagnostic Aspects

3.5.1 Ocular Signs

Decrease in tear secretion can be measured using a filter paper strip as described by Schirmer [23]. In the Schirmer-1 test, local anesthesia of the conjunctiva is not administered, whereas in the Schirmer-2 test it is. A result of less than 5 mm in 5 min is objective evidence of xerophthalmia, as defined by Vitali et al. (Table 3.1) [50].

The rose bengal test is used to establish a diagnosis of KCS. A value of more than 4 (on a scale of 9) is considered objective evidence of ocular dryness (Table 3.1).

3.5.2 Salivary Gland Involvement

3.5.2.1 Sialometry

In a group of patients with primary SS, 55% had abnormal parotid flow, while 88% had abnormal submandibular/sublingual flow [4]. According to the preliminary criteria of the European Study Group, the flow rate for unstimulated whole saliva should be measured, the flow being less than 1.5 ml in 15 min (Table 3.1). To obtain mean flow rates, at least two tests should be performed at about the same time of the day, on two different days. For the collection of saliva, the reader is referred to Sect. 1.3.1.

3.5.2.2 Sialochemistry

In a study in Israel, sodium, potassium, and immunoglobulin (Ig)A concentrations in saliva were significantly increased in patients with either primary or secondary SS [9].

3.5.2.3 Parotid Sialography

Sialography may or may not show ectasis; ductal changes are uncommon. In a Swedish study, sialographic changes appeared more often in the parotid than in the submandibular glands, but the most advanced changes were observed in the submandibular glands [26]. In a Japanese study of 107 patients suspected of having primary SS based on complaints of dry mouth and dry eyes, parotid sialography identified 37 patients with punctate ("apple tree in blossom"), globular, cavitary, or destructive sialectasia [37]. In another study, the presence of acinar dilatations and the disappearance of the homogeneous parenchymal "blush" were mentioned as the most relevant sialographic aspects in primary SS patients [27].

According to the European criteria, only the findings of *parotid* sialography are taken into account as objective evidence of salivary gland involvement. However, no specifications have been provided. In other words, the sialographic criteria have not been defined (Table 3.1).

3.5.2.4 Salivary Scintigraphy

Scintigraphy in patients suffering from SS may show a decrease in the uptake of the radioisotope in both the parotid and the submandibular glands. The most important finding is the failure of parotid or submandibular glands, or both, to empty in response to pilocarpine [3]. In other words, the salivary functional impairment in SS is shown by a decreased mean rate of excretion values. Based upon another study, it was concluded that salivary gland scintigraphy has only a limited discriminatory value for the diagnosis of primary SS [28]. Nevertheless, "salivary scintigraphy" is mentioned as one of the criteria of objective evidence of salivary gland involvement in the European criteria (Table 3.1). As with sialography, no criteria for the interpretation of scintigrams have been defined.

3.5.2.5 Biopsy of (Minor) Salivary Glands

Some authors have a preference for an open biopsy of the parotid gland for objective confirmation by histopathology of the diagnosis of

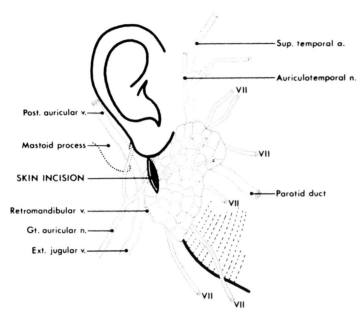

Fig. 3.2. Biopsy of parotid gland. (Reprinted with permission from [17])

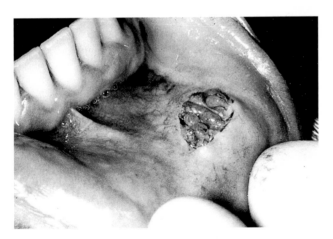

Fig. 3.3. Labial biopsy as a diagnostic procedure in Sjögren's syndrome. (Courtesy of Dr. T.E. Daniels, USA)

salivary inflammatory exocrinopathy (Fig. 3.2) [17]. Other authors prefer a biopsy of the sublingual gland [1]. However, the most common site for a biopsy in cases of suspected SS is the lower lip [13, 15]. The majority of the reports support the usefulness of such a biopsy for the diagnosis of SS (Fig. 3.3). Indeed, in the preliminary criteria for the classification of SS, only the findings of a minor salivary gland biopsy have been included (Table 3.1), mentioning a focus score of one or more per 4 mm² glandular tissue. Others have suggested that attention should be paid to the amount of glandular destruction [12].

The labial biopsy can easily be performed with local anesthesia. At least five lobules should be removed. Complications other than slight bleeding and temporarily reduced sensation do not occur if the lower lip is chosen as the biopsy site [35]. The histological aspects will be discussed below (see Sect. 3.6).

3.5.3 Autoantibodies

Serological studies for the detection of an associated autoimmune disease include a latex fixation test for rheumatoid factor, antinuclear antibody, and antibodies against SS-A (cytoplasmic proteins) and SS-B (nuclear proteins) [19]. Most patients have elevated total serum IgG [5, 6] and IgM-rheumatoid factor (RF) [29]. For the diagnosis of primary SS, only a positive anti-Ro/SS-A or anti-La/SS-B antibody serological finding is acceptable [50].

3.6 Histological Aspects

The histological features of the parotid glands in patients with SS may be similar to those seen in benign lymphoepithelial lesions or may merely show atrophy of the parenchyma.

The histological features of a labial gland biopsy are characterized by atrophy of the acini and replacement by lymphocytes (mainly CD4+ lymphocytes), the T helper cells [5]. Infiltrates are more prominent in the central portion of the lobule than in the periphery (Fig. 3.4). Several grading systems have been applied for quantification [53, 54]. A score of greater than one focus of at least 50 mononuclear cells

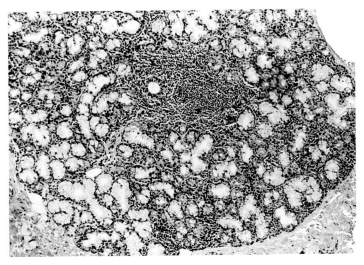

Fig. 3.4. Low-power view of salivary gland biopsy from lower lip, showing a focus of lymphocytes

per 4mm^2 glandular tissue, in the presence of an average of four evaluable lobules, is regarded as reliable and disease specific [50]. They are usually found next to small veins or ducts.

In a study of 113 patients who were suspected of having SS, periductal lymphocytic infiltration of the labial and/or parotid glands was observed in only 50% [36]. In a comparison of parotid and minor salivary gland biopsy for the diagnosis of SS, it was concluded that parotid gland biopsy adds very little to the labial salivary gland biopsy in the diagnosis of primary SS, but that parotid inflammatory changes may reflect disease duration and/or severity [55].

In a study comprising labial gland biopsies from 11 SS patients, a significant increase (more than 10% of the total plasma cell population) of IgM-positive plasma cells was found [43]. The authors speculated that patients with a high number of IgM-positive cells are at greater risk of developing lymphoma, in spite of a lack of evidence of monoclonality when staining for κ and λ light chains. Others have also used qualitative and quantitative analysis of plasma cells as diagnostic criteria [10, 53, 54]. However, others have suggested that changes in glandular plasma cell populations in SS are nonspecific [30].

In some patients with SS, either primary or secondary, the presence of Epstein-Barr virus (EBV) DNA in epithelial cells of acini and ducts of sublabial salivary glands has been demonstrated [41]. Among 14 patients with a non-Hodgkin's lymphoma that developed in SS, EBV DNA was detected in increased amounts in the tumor tissue of one patient [21]. However, in another study it has been shown that EBV DNA is commonly present in salivary glands [16].

Conjunctival biopsies in patients suffering from SS have been studied [31]. Metaplasia of the conjunctival epithelium was observed in all the patients, associated with a reduced number of goblet cells and a polymorphic inflammatory cell infiltrate of the stroma; the lymphocytic infiltrate was predominantly of the T cell type. In a study of the submandibular, labial, and lacrimal glands of 102 postmortem subjects, a wider than hitherto recognized spectrum of systemic inflammatory diseases was discovered to contribute to lymphocytic adenitis and degeneration of exocrine glands, requiring additional diagnostic tests for the diagnosis of SS [42]. Similar findings were reported in a study of 207 autopsy cases of patients who had no collagen diseases and in whom an age-related increase in focal lymphocytic infiltration in the submandibular glands was observed [25]; the same was true in the labial salivary glands [46].

3.7 Treatment and Prognosis

Treatment is usually symptomatic with regard to the dry mouth and the dry eyes. Sialogogues (substances that stimulate salivary production) are only useful in patients who still have functioning salivary tissue [5]. Mucin-containing lozenges seem to be preferable [22]. Pilocarpine, either in tablet form (2.5–5 mg three times daily) or as a 2% liquid ophthalmic solution (four drops three times a day as a swallowed mouth rinse for 6 weeks), has shown to be quite effective, particularly in patients with secondary SS [34]. Other workers have reported similar results [19]. Apparently, pilocarpine can be administered for up to 1 year without side effects (see also Chap. 1). Side effects encountered with excessive doses are sweating, nausea, and diarrhea [18]. In severe cases, administration of corticosteroids may be considered. In a 2-year double-blind crossover trial in 19 patients with primary SS, the use of hydroxychloroquine at a dose of 400 mg daily taken over a 12-month period did not have a worthwhile clinical benefit, despite improvement of hyperglobulinemia and slight changes in the erythrocyte sedimentation rate and IgM levels [24].

In cases of persistent bilateral parotid swelling, a conservative bilateral parotidectomy may be considered for esthetic reasons, with or without additional soft tissue reconstruction of the parotid region [48].

Patients with SS may have an increased risk of the development of non-Hodgkin's lymphoma [7]. Most of these lymphomas are of B cell origin, are of the mucosa-associated lymphoid tissue (MALT) type, and are centrocytic-like [14, 45]. Only a few cases of T cell non-Hodgkin's lymphoma have been reported [49]. At the same time, it should be realized that the distinction between malignant lymphoma and pseudolymphoma in patients with SS may lead to diagnostic difficulties [14].

Some authors have suggested the use of labial salivary gland biopsies to monitor the potential development of SS into pseudolymphoma and, finally, into malignant lymphoma [13]. The κ to λ ratio seems to be an important prognostic indicator [11, 44].

Approximately 70% of patients with SS and cutaneous vasculitis develop peripheral and/or central nervous system disease, probably also due to a vasculopathy [2].

References

1. Adam P, Haroun A, Billet J, et al. Biopsie des glandes salivaires. Intérêt et technique de la biopsie de la glande sublinguale sur sont versant antéro-latéral. Rev Stomatol Chir maxillofac 1992; 93: 337–340.
2. Alexander E, Provost TT. Sjögren's Syndrome. Association of cutaneous vasculitis with central nervous system disease. Arch Dermatol 1987; 123: 801–810.
3. Arrago JP, Rain JD, Brocheriou C, et al. Scintigraphy of the salivary glands in Sjögren's syndrome. J Clin Pathol 1987; 40: 1463–1467.
4. Atkinson JC, Travis WD, Pillemer SR, et al. Major salivary gland function in primary Sjögren's syndrome and its relationship to clinical features. J Rheumatol 1990; 17: 319–322.
5. Atkinson JC, Fox PC. Sjögren's syndrome: oral and dental considerations. JADA 1993; 124: 74–86.
6. Atkinson JC, Royce LS, Wellner R, et al. Anti-salivary antibodies in primary Sjögren's syndrome. J Oral Pathol Med 1995; 24: 206–212.

7. Batsakis JG. Primary lymphomas of the major salivary glands. Ann Otol Rhinol Laryngol 1986; 95: 107–108.

8. Baudet-Pommel M, Albuisson E, Kemeny L, et al. Early dental loss in Sjögren's syndrome. Histologic correlates. Oral Surg Oral Med Oral Pathol 1994; 78: 181–186.

9. Ben-Aryeh H, Spielman A, Szargel R, et al. Sialochemistry for diagnosis of Sjögren's syndrome in xerostomic patients. Oral Surg Oral Med Oral Pathol 1981; 52: 487–490.

10. Bodeutsch C, de Wilde PCM, Kater L, et al. Quantitative immunohistologic criteria are superior to the lymphatic focus score criterion for the diagnosis of Sjögren's syndrome. Arthritis Rheum 1992; 35: 1075–1087.

11. Bodeutsch C, de Wilde PCM, Kater L, et al. Monotypic plasma cells in labial salivary glands of patients with Sjögren's syndrome: Prognosticator for systemic lymphoproliferative disease. J Clin Pathol 1993; 46: 123–128.

12. Charpentier le Y, Auriol M. Qu'attendre de l'étude au microscope d'une biopsie de glandes salivaires accessoires (G.S.A.)? Rev Stomatol Chir maxillofac 1994; 95: 306–309.

13. Chomette G, Auriol M, Labrousse F, et al. Immunopathologie des glandes salivaires labiales dans le syndrome de Sjögren et les autres maladies dysimmunes. Rev Stomatol Chir maxillofac 1988; 89: 237–241.

14. Chomette G, Guilbert F, Auriol M, et al. Lymphomes des glandes salivaires. Frontières nosologiques nouvelles. Rev Stomatol Chir maxillofac 1990; 91 (suppl. 1): 32–35.

15. Daniels TE. Labial salivary gland biopsy in Sjögren's syndrome. Assessment as a diagnostic criterion in 326 suspected cases. Arthritis and Rheumatism 1984; 27: 147–156.

16. Deacon EM, Matthews JB, Potts AJC, et al. Detection of Epstein-Barr virus antigens and DNA in major and minor salivary glands using immunocytochemistry and polymerase chain reaction: possible relationship with Sjögren's syndrome. J Pathol 1991; 163: 351–360.

17. Ferguson JW, Edwards JL, Christmas PI, et al. Parotid gland biopsy for investigation of xerostomia. Br J Oral Maxillofac Surg 1990; 28: 234–237.

18. Ferguson MM. Pilocarpine and other cholinergic drugs in the management of salivary gland dysfunction. Oral Surg Oral Med Oral Pathol 1993; 75: 186–191.

19. Fox PC, Atkinson JC, Macynski AA, et al. Pilocarpine treatment of salivary gland hypofunction and dry mouth (xerostomia). Arch Intern Med 1991; 151: 1149–1152.

20. Fox RI. VIth International Symposium on Sjögren's Syndrome. Clinical aspects and therapy. Clinical Rheumatology 1995; 14 (suppl. 1): 17–19.

21. Fox RI, Luppi M, Kang H-I, et al. Reactivation of Epstein-Barr virus in Sjögren's syndrome. Springer Semin Immunopathol 1991; 13: 217–231.

22. Gravenmade EJ, Vissink A. Mucin-containing lozenges in the treatment of intraoral problems associated with Sjögren's syndrome. A double-blind cross-over study in 42 patients. Oral Surg Oral Med Oral Pathol 1993; 75: 466–471.

23. Hanson J, Fikentscher R, Roseburg R. Schirmer test of lacrimation. Its clinical importance. Arch Otolaryng 1975; 101: 293–295.

24. Kruize AA, Hené RJ, Kallenberg CGM, et al. Hydroxychloroquine treatment in primary Sjögren's syndrome: a two year double blind crossover trial. Ann Rheum Dis 1993; 52: 360–364.

25. Kurashima C, Hirokawa K. Age-related increase of focal lymphocytic infiltration in the human submandibular glands. J Oral Pathol Med 1986; 15: 172–178.

26. Lindvall AM, Jonsson R. The salivary gland component of Sjögren's syndrome: An evaluation of diagnostic methods. Oral Surg Oral Med Oral Pathol 1986; 62: 32–42.

27. Markusse HM, van Putten WIJ, Breedveld FC, et al. Digital subtraction sialography of the parotid glands in primary Sjögren's syndrome. J Rheumatol 1993; 20: 279–283.

28. Markusse HM, Pillay M, Breedveld FC. The diagnostic value of salivary gland scintigraphy in patients suspected of primary Sjögren's syndrome. Br J Rheumatol 1993; 32: 231–235.

29. Markusse HM, Oudkerk M, Vroom ThM, et al. Primary Sjögren's syndrome: clinical spectrum and mode of presentation based on an analysis of 50 patients selected from a department of rheumatology. Neth J Med 1992; 40: 125–134.

30. Matthews JB, Deacon EM, Wilson C, et al. Plasma cell populations in labial salivary glands from patients with and without Sjögren's syndrome. Histopathology 1993; 23: 399–407.

31. Raphael M, Bellefqih S, Piette JCh, et al. Conjunctival biopsy in Sjögren's syndrome: correlations between histological and immunohistochemical features. Histopathology 1988; 13: 191–202.

32. Reveille JD, Wilson RW, Provost TT, et al. Primary Sjögren's syndrome and other autoimmune diseases in families. Ann Intern Med 1984; 101: 748–756.

33. Rhodus NL, Colby S, Moller K, et al. Quantitative assessment of dysphagia in patients with primary and secondary Sjögren's syndrome. Oral Surg Oral Med Oral Pathol 1995; 79: 305–310.

34. Rhodus NL, Schuh MJ. Effects of pilocarpine on salivary flow in patients with Sjögren's syndrome. Oral Surg Oral Med Oral Pathol 1991; 72: 545–549.

35. Richards A, Mutlu S, Scully C, et al. Complications associated with labial salivary gland biopsy in the investigation of connective tissue disorders. Ann Rheumatic Dis 1992; 51: 996–997.

36. Saito T, Fukuda H, Arisue M, et al. Periductal lymphocytic infiltration of salivary glands in Sjögren's syndrome with relation to clinical and immunologic findings. Oral Surg Oral Med Oral Pathol 1991; 71: 179–183.

37. Saito T, Fukuda H, Arisue M, et al. Relationship between sialographic findings of parotid glands and histopathologic finding of labial glands in Sjögren's syndrome. Oral Surg Oral Med Oral Pathol 1991; 72: 675–680.

38. Saito T, Fukuda H, Takashi N, et al. Sjögren's syndrome in the adolescent. Report of four cases. Oral Surg Oral Med Oral Pathol 1994; 77: 368–372.

39. Sato T, Matsubara O, Tanaka Y, et al. Association of Sjögren's syndrome with pulmonary hypertension: report of two cases and review of the literature. Hum Pathol 1993; 24: 199–295.

40. Schi dt M, Dodd CL, Greenspan D, et al. Natural history of HIV-associated salivary gland disease. Oral Surg Oral Med Oral Pathol 1992; 74: 326–331.

41. Schuurman H-J, Schemman MHG, Weger de RA, et al. Epstein-Barr virus in the sublabial salivary gland in Sjögren's syndrome. Am J Clin Pathol 1989; 91: 461–463.
42. Segerberg-Konttinen M. Focal adenitis in lacrimal and salivary glands. A postmortem study. Scand J Rheumatology 1988; 17: 379–385.
43. Speight PM, Cruchley A, Williams DM. Quantification of plasma cells in labial salivary glands: increased expression of IgM in Sjögren's syndrome. J Oral Pathol Med 1990; 19: 126–130.
44. Speight PM, Jordan R, Colloby P, et al. Early detection of lymphomas in Sjögren's syndrome by *in situ* hybridisation for k and light chain mRNA in labial salivary glands. Oral Oncol, Eur J Cancer 1994; 30B: 244–247.
45. Stewart A, Blenkinsopp PT, Henry K. Bilateral parotid MALT lymphoma and Sjögren's syndrome. Br J Oral Maxillfoac Surg 1994; 32: 318–322.
46. Takeda Y, Komori A. Focal lymphocytic infiltration in the human labial salivary glands: a postmortem study. J Oral Pathol Med 1986; 15: 83–86.
47. Terada K, Katamine S, Eguchi K, et al. Prevalence of serum and salivary antibodies to HTLV-1 in Sjögren's syndrome. Lancet 1994; 344: 1116–1119.
48. Timosca GH. Résultats à long terme des parotidectomies totales bilatérales dans le syndrome de Sjögren. Rev Stomatol Chir maxillofac 1994; 95: 133–135.
49. Valk van der PGM, Hollema H, van Voorst vander PC, et al. Sjögren's syndrome with specific cutaneous manifestations and multifocal clonal T-cell populations progressing to a cutaneous pleomorphic T-cell lymphoma. Am J Clin Pathol 1989; 92: 357–361.
50. Vitali C, Bombardieri S, Moutsopoulos HM, et al. Preliminary criteria for the classification of Sjögren's syndrome. Results of a prospective concerted action supported by the European Community. Arthritis and Rheumatism 1993; 36: 340–347.
51. Wang SL, Zou ZJ, Yu SF, et al. Recurrent swelling of parotid glands and Sjögren's syndrome. Int J Oral Maxillofac Surg 1993; 22: 362–365.
52. Warfvinge G, Larsson A, Henricsson V, et al. Salivary gland involvement in autoimmune thyroiditis, with special reference to the degree of association with Sjögren's syndrome. Oral Surg Oral Med Oral Pathol 1992; 74: 288–293.
53. Wilde de PCM, Baak JPA, Houwelingen van JC, et al. Morphometric study of histological changes in sublabial salivary glands due to aging process. J Clin Pathol 1986; 39: 406–417.
54. Wilde de PCM, Baak JPA, Slootweg PJ, et al. Morphometry in the diagnosis of Sjögren's syndrome. Analytical and Quantitative Cytology and Histology 1986; 8: 49–55.
55. Wise CM, Agudelo CA, Semble EL, et al. Comparison of parotid and minor salivary gland biopsy in the diagnosis of Sjögren's syndrome. Arthritis Rheum 1988; 31: 662–666.

4 Cysts

4.1 Cysts of Major Salivary Glands

Cysts in the major salivary glands are rare. Occasionally, a lymphoepithelial cyst or a salivary duct cyst may be encountered in these glands. Lymphoepithelial cysts and branchial cysts appear to share a common element, namely the inclusion of ductal tissue within a lymph node matrix [19]. Polycystic (dysgenetic) bilateral disease of the parotid glands is rare.

4.1.1 Lymphoepithelial Cyst

Brocheriou et al. [7] classify parotid gland cysts as developmental (dysgenetic) cysts and acquired cysts. Among the developmental cysts, the lymphoepithelial cyst, also referred to as the branchial cyst, is the most common type. The lymphoepithelial cyst is thought to develop by cystic degeneration of epithelial salivary cells that have been enclosed in intraparotid or paraparotid lymph nodes. Malignant transformation is very uncommon [12].

The clinical presentation is of a localized, cystic lesion. Unilateral and bilateral cystic lesions of the parotid glands have also been reported in human immunodeficiency virus (HIV)-infected patients. These lesions have been shown to represent lymphoepithelial cysts (see also Chap. 6). Histologically, the lumen of the lymphoepithelial cyst is lined by squamous epithelium with varying amounts of lymphoid tissue.

Treatment usually requires a (superficial) parotidectomy.

4.1.2 Polycystic (Dysgenetic) Disease of the Parotid Glands

Only a few cases of polycystic (dysgenetic) disease of the parotid glands have been reported. Batsakis et al. [5] listed the following features, based on three cases from the literature and three cases from their own files:

1. The disease only occurs in females.
2. There is almost always bilateral involvement.
3. Patients have a history of fluctuating, nontender parotid gland swelling for several years.
4. Sialograms show cystic changes of the main parotid duct.

Two cases have been reported with a confirmed familial background [18].

The histological features are characterized by a honeycomb appearance, with minimal or no signs of inflammation. The disease may be misdiagnosed histologically as carcinoma.

Superficial parotidectomy appears to be the most suitable surgical approach, if indicated for diagnostic or cosmetic reasons. However, enlargement of the cysts in the deep lobe may lead to a subsequent clinical recurrence [18].

4.1.3 Salivary Duct Cyst

The rare salivary duct cyst probably occurs as result of obstruction in the majority of cases and is more or less limited to the parotid gland; occurrence in the submandibular gland is very uncommon [20].

Patients are usually above 40 years of age. Clinically, the salivary duct cyst can not be distinguished from the lymphoepithelial cyst [3, 4] (Fig. 4.1).

Histologically, the cyst wall is lined by a single- or multilayered columnar, cuboidal, or squamous epithelium [2]. Goblet cells may be present.

Treatment usually requires a (superficial) parotidectomy.

4.2 Cysts of Minor Salivary Glands

Cystic lesions of the minor salivary glands are usually not considered to be true cysts, something which is reflected in terms such as "mucous escape reaction" and "mucous retention phenomenon."

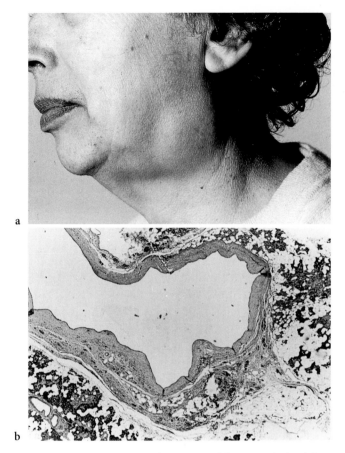

Fig. 4.1. **a** Cystic lesion in lower part of the parotid gland. **b** Low-power view of the surgical specimen shows the salivary duct cyst in the superficial lobe

4.2.1 Definition

The mucous retention phenomenon (MRP), also called mucous cyst or sialocyst, refers to the retention of mucous. Some authors use the term "mucous escape reaction" or "mucous retention cyst," depending on an epithelial lining is absent or present [14]. Some authors recognize three subtypes of oral sialocysts [9]: (1) true mucous retention cyst, (2) reactive oncocytoid cyst, and (3) mucopapillary cyst.

4.2.2 Etiology

MRP is most likely caused by obstruction or traumatic severance of the excretory ducts, in some instances as the result of previous surgery.

4.2.3 Epidemiology

MRP occurs at all ages, without any preference for either men or women. Congenital occurrence is very unusual [1].

4.2.4 Clinical Aspects

MRP mainly occurs as a solitary lesion in the minor salivary glands of the lower lip; multiple occurrence is rare [16]. The floor of the mouth is another site of predilection. Mucous retention in other oral locations is rare.

When the lower lip is involved, the term *mucocele* is used. The cyst appears as a soft, bluish swelling and usually measures less than 1 cm (Fig. 4.2). The swelling may be of recurrent nature, but is otherwise asymptomatic. The history and clinical aspect are more or less

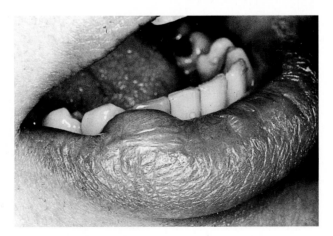

Fig. 4.2. Mucocele of the lower lip

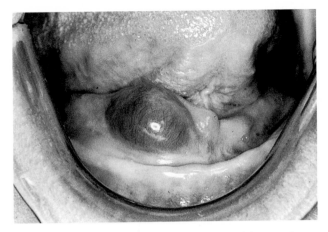

Fig. 4.3. Bluish appearing ranula in the floor of the mouth

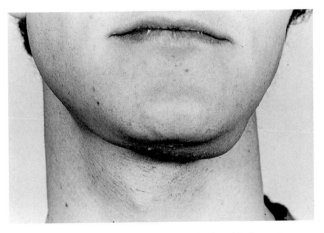

Fig. 4.4. Submental swelling caused by "plunging" ranula

pathognomic, since other cysts or neoplasms in the lower lip are rare. It is almost unheard of for a mucocele to be located in the upper lip, as most localized swellings of the upper lip are salivary gland neoplasms or other types of neoplasms.

When located in the floor of the mouth, the term *ranula* is used. ("Rana" is the Latin word for "frog"). Typically, the sublingual gland is the secretory source. A ranula may reach a considerable size, occupying one or both sides of the floor of the mouth (Fig. 4.3). Cystic tumors of the sublingual gland, though extremely rare, may clinically mimic a ranula.

In rare instances, there is an extension of a ranula through the mylohyoid muscle, resulting in a submental or submandibular swelling, also referred to as plunging ranula (Fig. 4.4). Bilateral occurrence of a plunging ranula is rare. It may be difficult to make a preoperative diagnosis of plunging ranula if there is no clinically evident connection between the floor of the mouth and the submental or submandibular swelling. In such cases, the injection of 0.5 ml contrast-medium, e.g. Lipiodol (iodized oil), into the sublingual space can be considered. If the contrast medium extends into the neck on radiography, it indicates a plunging ranula [21]. A simpler diagnostic aid in this situation is fine-needle aspiration cytology.

4.2.5 Histological Aspects

Histopathologic examination of the lesion shows a well-circumscribed or a diffusely spread pool of mucous, either surrounded by a wall of granulation tissue or, quite rarely, by an epithelial lining (Fig. 4.5). The type of epithelial lining varies from

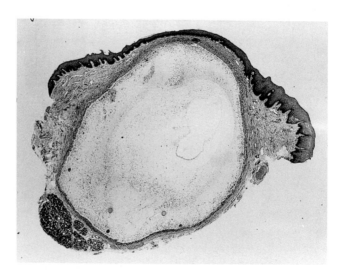

Fig. 4.5. Low-power view of a mucocele of the lower lip

cuboidal to columnar or squamous cell epithelium and may represent the lining of a preexisting, dilated excretory duct. In such cases, the term "mucous retention phenomenon, retention type" may be used, whereas in the absence of such an epithelial lining the term "mucous retention phenomenon, extravasation type" is used. In cases of long duration, the mucous content may be replaced by immature connective tissue. Fibrosis will eventually occur.

Superficially located mucous cysts may be confused with vesiculobullous disease, both clinically and histologically [13].

Occasionally, confusion arises with regard to the distinction between a mucocele and an acinic cell carcinoma. Acinic cells usually stain negative for mucin and show periodic acid-Schiff (PAS) positivity, whereas the foamy histiocytes in a mucocele usually stain positive for mucin and do not react to PAS staining.

4.2.6 Treatment

Although a mucous retention cyst is a harmless phenomenon that may regress after secondary traumatization, e.g., biting, recurrences are common, necessitating surgical removal. Many patients request surgical removal for cosmetic reasons. Ranulas usually cause discomfort and also require surgical treatment.

It is almost always possible to remove a mucocele of the lower lip by an excisional biopsy using local anesthesia. Part of the overlying mucosa should be included in order to prevent rupture of the cyst. The adjacent salivary gland lobules may be removed as well. Primary closure can easily be obtained in this location. Healing is usually uneventful, and recurrences are rare. In a small series of 18 patients, effective treatment with cryosurgery, without anesthesia, has been reported [22].

Treatment of a ranula is more difficult because of the larger size and the more complex anatomy of the floor of the mouth. In some cases, particularly in the presence of an epithelial lining, it is sufficient to marsupialize the lesion by simply removing the upper part together with the overlying mucosa [8]. Packing the entire pseudocystic cavity with gauze minimizes the rate of recurrence [6]. In lesions less than 1 cm in diameter, excision may be attempted rather than marsupialization. In the case of recurrence or persistence, the ipsilateral sublingual gland should be removed. Some authors advocate the removal of the sublingual gland together with the ranula [26].

When dealing with a plunging ranula, removal of the sublingual gland usually suffices, making it unnecessary to attempt to remove the entire lesion [25]. For the removal of the sublingual gland, an incision in the floor of the mouth directly over the gland can be made. Canulation of the submandibular duct is recommended for reasons of identification and protection. Some authors prefer to approach the sublingual gland by raising a mucoperiosteal flap from the medial surface of the mandible [10].

4.3 Intraosseous Cyst of Possible Salivary Gland Origin

A few cases have been reported of an intraosseous jaw cyst that showed histological features of salivary gland origin, such as the presence of mucin and salivary tissue [11, 17, 23, 24]. Furthermore, there is some resemblance to the so-called mucoepidermoid carcinoma. In view of the small number of reported cases, it has not yet been determined whether the *sialo-odontogenic cyst*, also referred to as the glandular odontogenic cyst, does in fact represent a separate entity. Nevertheless, this cyst is included in the WHO classification of odontogenic tumors [15].

References

1. Addante RR. Congentical cystic dilatation of the submandibular duct. Oral Surg Oral Med Oral Pathol 1984; 58: 656–658.
2. Altman K, Bailey BMW. Parotid cyst: a case report. Int J Oral Maxillofac Surg 1994; 23: 165–166.
3. Antoniades K, Karakasis D, Tzarou V, et al. Benign cysts of the parotid gland. Int J Oral Maxillofac Surg 1990; 19: 139–140.
4. Assimakopoulos D, Malamou-Mitsi V, Skevas A. Notre expérience des kystes de la parotide. Rev Stomatol Chir maxillofac 1995; 96: 313–316.
5. Batsakis JG, Bruner JM, Luna MA. Polycystic (dysgenetic) disease of the parotid glands. Arch Otolaryngol Head Neck Surg 1988; 114: 1146–1148.
6. Baurmash HD. Marsupialization for treatment of oral ranula: a second look at the procedure. J Oral Maxillofac Surg 1992; 50: 1274–1279.
7. Brocheriou C, Laufer J, de Roquancourt A, et al. Kystes et pseudo-kystes de la parotide. Rev Stomatol Chir maxillofac 1990; 91: 281–285.

8. Crysdale WS, Mendelsohn JD, Conley S. Ranulas – mucoceles of the oral cavity: experience in 26 children. Laryngoscope 1988; 98: 296–298.

9. Eversole LR. Oral sialocysts. Arch Otolaryngol Head Neck Surg 1987; 113: 51–56.

10. Galloway RH, Gross PD, Thompson SH, et al. Pathogenesis and treatment of ranula: Report of three cases. J Oral Maxillofac Surg 1989; 47: 299–302.

11. Gardner DG, Kessler HP, Morency R, et al. The glandular odontogenic cyst: an apparent entity. J Oral Pathol 1988; 17: 359–366.

12. Hill S, Francis N, Thomas JM. Primary carcinoma arising in a lympho-epithelial cyst of the parotid gland. Eur J Surg Oncol 1994; 20: 164–164.

13. Jensen JL. Superficial mucoceles of the oral mucosa. Am J Dermatopathol 1990; 12: 88–92.

14. Koudelka BM, Obstructive disorders. In: Surgical Pathology of the salivary glands. Ellis GL, Auclair PL, Gnepp DR (eds.). W.B. Saunders Comp., Philadelphia-Tokyo, 1991.

15. Kramer IRH, Pindborg JJ, Shear M. WHO International Classification of Tumours. Histological Typing of Odontogenic Tumours. 2nd ed. Springer-Verlag; Berlin, Heidelberg, New York, 1992.

16. McCaul JA, Lamey P-J. Multiple oral mucoceles treated with gamma-linolenic acid: report of a case. Br J Oral Maxillofac Surg 1994; 32: 392–393.

17. Padayachee A, Van Wyk, CW. Two cystic lesions with features of both the botryoid odontogenic cyst and the central mucoepidermoid tumor: Sialo-odontogenic cyst? J Oral Pathol Med 1987; 16: 499–504.

18. Smyth AG, Ward-Booth RP, High AS. Polycystic disease of the parotid glands: two familial cases. Br J Oral Maxillofac Surg 1993; 31: 38–40.

19. Som PM, Brandwein MS, Silvers A. Nodal inclusion cysts of the parotid gland and parapharyngeal space: a discussion of lymphohepithelial, AIDS-related parotid, and branchial cysts, cystic Warthin's tumors, and cysts in Sjögren's syndrome. Laryngoscope 1995; 105: 1122–1128.

20. Surkin M, Remsen K, Lawson W, et al. A mucocele of the submandibular gland. Arch Otolaryngol 1985; 111: 623–625.

21. Takimoto T. Radiograpic technique for preoperative diagnosis of plunging ranula. J Oral Maxillofac Surg 1991; 49: 659.

22. Toida M, Ishimaru J-I, Hobo N. A simple cryosurgical method for treatment of oral mucous cysts. Int J Oral Maxillofac Surg 1993; 22; 353–355.

23. Toida M, Nakashima E, Okumura Y, et al. Glandular odontogenic cyst: a case report and literature review. J Oral Maxillofac Surg 1994; 52: 1312–1316.

24. Vesper M, Günzl H-J, Hellner D, et al. Die sialo-odontogene (glandulär-odontogene) Zyste. Klinisch-pathologische Analyse von 3 Fällen und Literaturübersicht. Dtsch Z Mund Kiefer GesichtsChir 1994; 18: 254–256.

25. Visscher de JGAM, Wal van der KGH, Vogel de PL. The plunging ranula. Pathogenesis, diagnosis and management. J Cranio-Max-Fac Surg 1989; 17: 182–185.

26. Yoshimura Y, Obara S, Kondoh T, et al. A comparison of three methods used for treatment of ranula. J Oral Maxillofac Surg 1995; 53: 280–282.

5 Neoplasms

5.1 Introduction

The majority of primary neoplasms of salivary glands in adults are of epithelial origin, being derived from parenchymal cells. In children, *hemangiomas* and *lymphangiomas* are the dominant tumors in the parotid gland [131]. *Hemangiopericytomas* of the parotid gland are rare [120], as are glomus tumors [164].

In a series of 178 *mesenchymal* salivary gland tumors, accounting for 5% of all tumors of the salivary glands, angiomas and lipomas were the most common benign tumors, while only 21 sarcomas were observed [167]. Sarcomas are rare and mainly comprise malignant schwannomas, malignant fibrous histiocytomas, and fibrosarcomas [12, 130]. A few cases of intraparotid nodular fasciitis [71] and a case of primary malignant melanoma in the parotid gland have been reported [210].

Non-Hodgkin's lymphoma may occur in the parotid glands. It is not uncommon for it to be the only manifestation of the disease [105, 186]. Like other lymphomas of mucosa-associated lymphoid tissue, to which they bear a striking resemblance, salivary gland lymphomas may remain localized for prolonged periods with a tendency toward local recurrence rather than to distant spread. These properties may be explained by the histogenesis of these tumors from centrocyte-like cells that appear to be of similar lineage to splenic marginal zone cells [105]. Approximately 15% of malignant lymphomas of the salivary gland are *Hodgkin's lymphomas*. Extramedullary plasmacytomas in salivary glands are rare [62].

A few cases of *malignant salivary gland neoplasms* in the parotid gland have been reported after successful treatment of a primary malignant neoplasm elsewhere in the body, e.g., leukemia [126].

Occasionally, the major salivary glands are the site of a *metastatic tumor*. The parotid gland is the salivary gland most often involved in secondary deposits. Secondary neoplastic involvement of the major salivary glands can be from regional (supraclavicular) and distant (infraclavicular) primary neoplasms. Cutaneous squamous cell carcinomas and melanomas are the most frequent primary neoplasms of the former category, while carcinomas of the lungs, breast, and kidneys are the most frequent infraclavicular neoplasms that metastatize to the major salivary glands [25]. The infraclavicular neoplasms most often disseminate hematogenously.

This chapter will focus on the epithelial salivary gland neoplasms.

5.2 Etiology and Histogenesis

The etiology of epithelial salivary gland neoplasms is unknown. In occasional patients, there is a previous history of low-dose irradiation of the head and neck area, sometimes more than 20 years ago. The incidence of salivary gland tumors among those exposed in Hiroshima City was 20 times higher than among those not exposed [183]. In a study in Los Angeles, it was demonstrated that 28% of malignant parotid tumors were attributable to exposure of the parotid gland to diagnostic and therapeutic radiation [160]. In another study, no correlation was found between radon levels and the incidence of salivary gland neoplasms [143].

The possible association between breast carcinoma and salivary gland neoplasms and also between cutaneous neoplasms and salivary gland carcinoma has been another subject of debate [1, 142, 182]. It has been inferred that the salivary gland may be a hormone-dependent gland and that estrogen metabolism may occur in salivary glands and may therefore play a causative role in the development of these neoplasms [58].

There is evidence for a multicellular theory of epithelial salivary gland tumor histogenesis; in other words, any of the multiplicity of cell types in normal salivary glands have the potential to give rise to any of the various types of tumor occurring in this organ [53].

5.3 Epidemiology

In most parts of the world, the incidence of benign and malignant epithelial tumors of all salivary glands varies from 1–2 per 100000 per year. Unusual familial clustering of salivary gland carcinoma has been reported among the Eskimo population in Greenland [139].

There is no sex predominance for salivary gland neoplasms, nor is there a distinct racial preference [66]. Patients of all ages can be affected. The majority of patients, however, are diagnosed between the fourth and seventh decade.

In several series of epithelial salivary gland tumors in children, the mucoepidermoid carcinoma was the most common malignant lesion [42, 72]. An exceptional entity is the benign congenital salivary gland tumor, also referred to as sialoblastoma, embryoma, or congenital epithelial tumor of the parotid gland [28, 101]. Histologically, there may be a strong resemblance to adenoid cystic carcinoma (ACC). Furthermore, there is also an entity known as "salivary gland anlage tumor" or "congenital pleomorphic adenoma"; it occurs at birth or within the first few days or weeks of life in the form of a polypoid lesion of the nasopharynx, causing respiratory distress [56].

5.4 Clinical Aspects

The majority of tumors occur in the parotid gland with just a small proportion located in the other glands, the distribution ratio being as follows: parotid gland to submandibular gland to sublingual gland to intraoral glands, 100:10:1:10.

As far as the character of the tumor is concerned, it should be observed that approximately 25% of parotid gland tumors are malignant, while the percentages for the submandibular, sublingual, and intraoral glands are 35%, almost 100%, and 50% or more, respectively.

5.4.1 Parotid Gland

5.4.1.1 Symptoms

The history may reveal a slow-growing tumor of many years' duration (Fig. 5.1). Rapid growth, pain, and facial paralysis are indicative of a

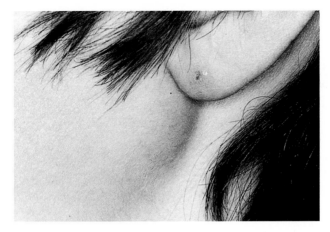

Fig. 5.1. Fairly typical presentation of parotid gland neoplasm

malignant tumor. In the absence of these symptoms, however, a malignant salivary gland tumor may still be present. Occasionally, inflammatory disease may clinically mimic a neoplasm [207]. In the submandibular gland, the term Küttner tumor is usually applied for these cases.

In rare instances, patients with a parotid gland neoplasm present with a temporomandibular joint problem [161]. On the other hand, cysts and tumors of the ascending ramus of the mandible may mimic a lesion of the parotid gland. This also holds true for a pilomatrixoma of the skin in the parotid region [208].

5.4.1.2 Clinical Findings

On palpation, the consistency of an epithelial salivary gland neoplasm may vary from cystic to firm and elastic. The tumor is usually freely movable from the skin and the underlying structures. Facial nerve impairment and pain are ominous signs; however, the absence of such symptoms does not rule out the possibility of a malignant salivary gland neoplasm.

The majority of parotid tumors are located lateral to the facial nerve. At times, it may be difficult to clinically evaluated whether the tumor is in the superficial or deep lobe. Limited mobility and diffuse swelling point to location in the deep lobe, as does bulging of the pharyngeal wall. Computed tomography (CT) may be a helpful aid in this matter [118].

Multifocality is rare. A small number of synchronous unilateral parotid neoplasms of different histological types have been reported [166]. A limited number of cases of bilateral salivary gland neoplasms other than Warthin tumor have been described [86]. Recurrent pleomorphic adenoma of the parotid gland often occurs in a multinodular fashion (Fig. 5.2).

Approximately 75% of parotid gland tumors are benign; of these, the commonest tumor is pleomorphic adenoma, previously called a mixed tumor.

The history and the clinical findings of a parotid swelling are often more or less sufficient for making a provisional diagnosis of a salivary gland neoplasm. At the same time, there are substantial risks in performing a (superficial) parotidectomy on the basis of a clinical diagnosis alone. Aspiration cytology is the most useful technique to obtain a more reliable preoperative diagnosis (see also Sect. 5.4.2).

5.4.2 Submandibular Gland

Approximately 10% of all salivary gland tumors are located in the submandibular glands, and 65% of these are benign, at least in West-

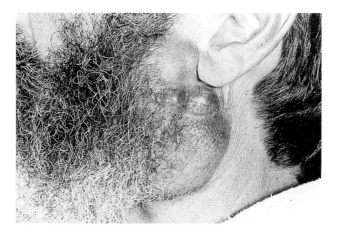

Fig. 5.2. Recurrent pleomorphic adenoma of parotid gland

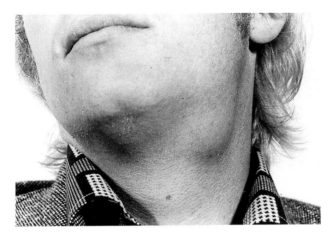

Fig. 5.3. Clinical presentation of submandibular gland neoplasm

ern countries. Submandibular tumors are apparently less likely to be malignant in some African countries.

Among the malignant salivary gland tumors of the submandibular gland, ACC and mucoepidermoid carcinoma are the commonest types. Pain and paralysis of the tongue may indicate spread of the tumor cells into the lingual and hypoglossal nerves. Otherwise, the clinical features and the history are similar to those described for neoplasms in the parotid gland (Fig. 5.3).

The most common error made in the preoperative clinical diagnosis of a neoplasm of the submandibular gland is the assumption that one is dealing with chronic sialoadenitis. Fine-needle aspiration cytology (FNAC) may be very helpful to avoid this pitfall.

The submandibular gland has a much higher attenuation value than the parotid gland, making it necessary to use a contrast medium in CT scans.

5.4.3 Sublingual Gland

Neoplasms of the sublingual gland are rare. Patients present with a submucosal swelling in the floor of the mouth (Fig. 5.4). Almost all of these neoplasms are malignant, although the neoplasm may be of long duration.

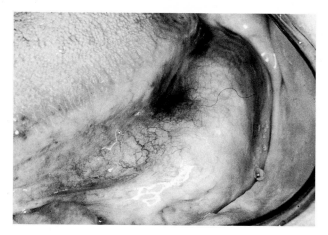

Fig. 5.4. Clinical presentation of salivary gland neoplasm arising from sublingual salivary gland, most likely a malignant type

5.4.4 Intraoral Salivary Gland

Approximately 10% of all salivary gland tumors are located in the intraoral, minor salivary glands. Fifty percent or more of these neoplasms are malignant [203]. With the possible exception of Warthin tumor, the same type of neoplasms may be encountered in the minor accessory glands as in the major glands.

The junction of the hard and soft palate is the most favored location for a neoplasm of minor salivary glands, followed by the upper lip (Figs. 5.5–5.8) [64]. The lower lip, the cheek mucosa, and the tongue are rare locations. In a series of 103 tumors of the lips, 87 were on the upper lip and 16 on the lower lip. Of the 87 on the upper lip all but a few were benign, while 15 of the 16 lower-lip tumors were found to be malignant [150].

The duration of salivary gland tumors of the intraoral salivary glands varies from several months to many years. In general, these neoplasms are asymptomatic, even the malignant ones [180]. Ulceration of the overlying mucosa is rare. Probably because of their long duration and their clinically inconspicuous nature, the possibility of a salivary gland neoplasm is rarely included in the clinical differential diagnosis of an intraoral swelling.

A biopsy should be taken in palatal salivary gland tumors, since the histological type may influence the extent of the surgical treatment. Other types of neoplasms may occur at the palate, such as (amelanotic) melanomas and non-Hodgkin's lymphomas.

In many cases, the biopsy specimen permits a reliable diagnosis to be made of the type of salivary gland tumor. In some cases, however,

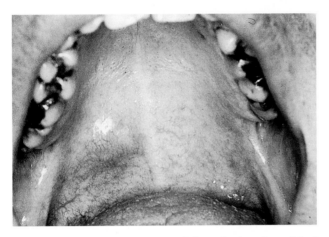

Fig. 5.5. Inconspicious-looking nodule at the junction of the hard and soft palate, suggestive of a salivary gland neoplasm, either benign or malignant

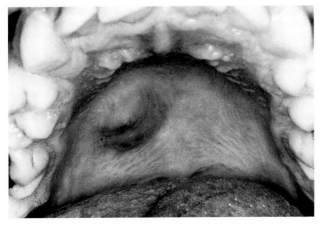

Fig. 5.6. Cystlike swelling of the palate caused by adenocarcinoma of salivary gland origin

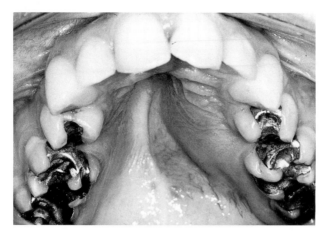

Fig. 5.7. Unilateral palatal swelling caused by adenoid cystic carcinoma

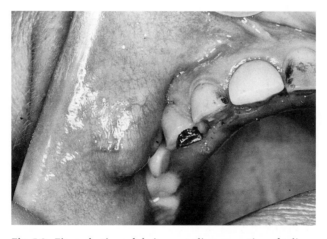

Fig. 5.8. Firm, elastic nodule in upper lip, suggestive of salivary gland neoplasm

the final diagnosis can only be made after examination of the whole surgical specimen.

In a small series of patients, magnetic resonance imaging (MRI) findings correlated well with the histopathologic findings [111].

5.4.5 Tumors in Other Sites

In rare instances, salivary gland tumors are located within the jaw bones, most frequently in the mandible (Figs. 5.9, 5.10). The

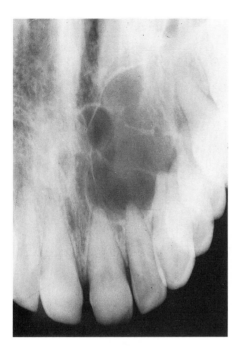

Fig. 5.9. Intraosseous mucoepidermoid carcinoma in the maxilla

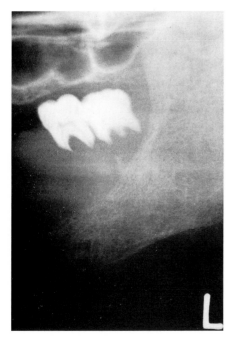

Fig. 5.10. Intraosseous spread of adenoid cystic carcinoma, producing a picture of teeth "floating in the air." (Courtesy of Dr. K.G.H. van der Wal, Netherlands)

mucoepidermoid carcinoma is the most common central salivary gland tumor reported in the literature [35, 37]. It is not always possible to be sure whether such a tumor has arisen primarily inside the bone or has spread into the bone from the surrounding soft tissues. Furthermore, the pathogenesis of intraosseous salivary gland neoplasms may be explained on the basis of metaplasia of odontogenic epithelium.

Salivary gland tumors in the area of the maxillary tuberosity probably originate from the maxillary sinus in most instances.

Because of the relatively small numbers of reported cases, there is no staging system for central salivary gland tumors, although a proposal has recently been made [36].

Occurrence of glandular tumors at other sites such as the external auditory canal, the middle ear, the larynx, the lacrimal glands, and the nasal cavity and paranasal sinuses is rare and will not be discussed here. The same applies to gingival salivary gland choristoma [34].

5.5 TNM Staging

A TNM staging system for malignant neoplasms of the major salivary glands is presented in Table 5.1.

Table 5.1. TNM Clinical Classification [98]

T	**Primary tumor**
TX	Primary tumor cannot be assessed
T0	No evidence of primary tumor
T1	Tumor 2 cm or less in greatest dimension
T2	Tumor more than 2 cm but not more than 4 cm in greatest dimension
T3	Tumor more than 4 cm but not more than 6 cm in greatest dimension
T4a	Tumor more than 6 cm in greatest dimension

Note: All categories are subdivided: (a) no local extension, (b) local extension. Local extension is clinical or macroscopic evidence of invasion of skin, soft tissues, bone, or nerve. Microscopic evidence alone is not local extension for classification purposes

N	**Regional lymph nodes**
NX	Regional lymph nodes cannot be assessed
N0	No regional lymph node metastasis
N1	Metastasis in a single ipsilateral lymph node, 3 cm or less in greatest dimension

Table 5.1. *Continued*

N2   Metastasis in a single ipsilateral lymph node, more than 3 cm but not more
          than 6 cm in greatest dimension, or in multiple ipsilateral lymph nodes,
          none more than 6 cm in greatest dimension, or in bilateral or
          contralateral lymph nodes, none more than 6 cm in greatest dimension
N2a   Metastasis in a single ipsilateral lymph node, more than 3 cm but not more
          than 6 cm in greatest dimension
N2b   Metastasis in multiple ipsilateral lymph nodes, none more than 6 cm in
          greatest dimension
N2c   Metastasis in bilateral or contralateral lymph nodes, none more than 6 cm
          in greatest dimension
N3   Metastasis in a lymph node more than 6 cm in greatest dimension
Note: Midline nodes are considered ipsilateral nodes

M   Distant metastasis
MX   Presence of distant metastasis cannot be assessed
M0   No distant metastasis
M1   Distant metastasis

pTNM Pathological Classification
The pT, pN, and pM categories correspond to the T, N, and M categories

Staging grouping

Stage I	T1a	N0	M0
	T2a	N0	M0
Stage II	T1b	N0	M0
	T2b	N0	M0
	T3a	N0	M0
Stage III	T3b	N0	M0
	T4a	N0	M0
	Any T (except T4b)	N1	M0
Stage IV	T4b	Any N	M0
	Any T	N2, N3	M0
	Any T	Any N	M1

Salivary glands
T1 ≤ 2 cm
T2 > 2–4 cm   Categories divided:
T3 > 4–6 cm   (a) no extension
T4 > 6 cm   (b) extension
N1 Ipsilateral single ≤3 cm
N2 Ipsilateral single >3–6 cm
    Ipsilateral multiple ≤6 cm
    Bilateral, contralateral ≤6 cm
N3 > 6 cm

5.6 Imaging Techniques

In most parts of the world, imaging techniques are not routinely used in the preoperative assessment of a salivary gland tumor. In selected cases, however, sialography (Fig. 5.11) and scintigraphy (Fig. 5.12) can be helpful diagnostic tools. The same applies to CT scans (Fig. 5.13), ultrasonographic examination (Fig. 5.14) [4, 32], and MRI [40, 41, 193]. MRI is claimed to be superior to CT for imaging parotid tumors, particularly in the case of recurrences [21, 40, 152]. Positron emission tomography (PET) was shown to be less useful in preoperative differentiation between malignant and benign neoplasms in 26 patients with parotid masses [135].

In general, an open biopsy of the parotid gland should be avoided because of possible damage to branches of the facial nerve and because of the chance of seeding tumor cells into the surrounding healthy tissues when dealing with a benign or malignant neoplasm. In other words, when considering the possibility of a neoplasm, a biopsy in the parotid region usually requires a (superficial) parotidectomy.

It is not necessary to use all of the diagnostic tools mentioned above. Clinicians should make their choice based on their own experience and the available expertise. In general, FNAC is the diagnostic tool of first choice.

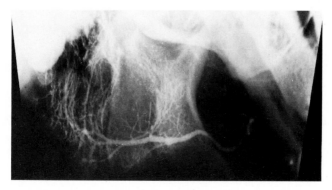

Fig. 5.11. Sialogram of benign (expansile) neoplasm of parotid gland

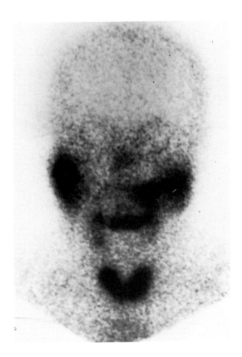

Fig. 5.12. Scintigram showing increased activity of right parotid gland due to the presence of a Warthin tumor

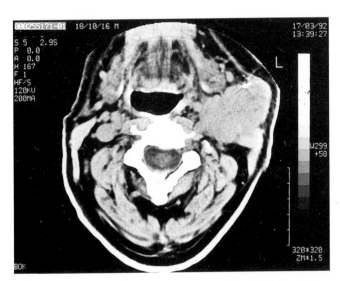

Fig. 5.13. Computed tomography (CT) scan of malignant neoplasm of left parotid gland extending caudally. (Courtesy of Dr. J.A. Castelijns, Netherlands)

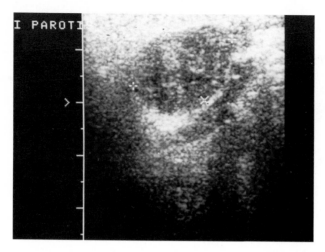

Fig. 5.14. Ultrasound picture of Warthin tumor in the superficial lobe of the parotid gland; note the low and slightly inhomogeneous echogeneity. (Courtesy of Dr. J.A. Castelijns, Netherlands)

5.7 Cytological Aspects

The value of preoperative FNAC lies mainly in the possibility it offers of distinguishing a salivary gland disorder from other pathologic conditions, e.g., lymphoreticular disease and metastatic deposits [70, 215]. In many, but not all instances, even the exact type of salivary gland tumor can be determined by FNAC (Fig. 5.15) [107]. A conservative attitude toward FNAC of the salivary glands will still provide considerable, safe diagnostic information for the benefit of both patient and clinician; while most common benign and malignant lesions can be accurately and precisely diagnosed, the not inconsiderable problems of interpretation should not be underestimated [213].

5.8 Histological Aspects

In this paragraph, discussion on the histopathology will be limited to the epithelial salivary gland tumors and is primarily based on the

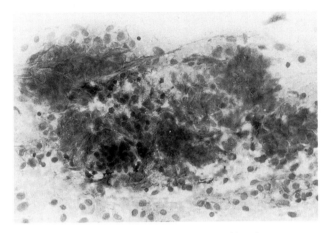

Fig. 5.15. Cytologic appearance of pleomorphic adenoma

histological typing of salivary tumors by the WHO in 1991 [168–170] (Table 5.2).

Almost any type of benign and malignant salivary gland neoplasm may demonstrate tumor-associated lymphoid infiltration, which may lead to misinterpretation as metastatic disease [13]. Based on a small series of patients, it has been claimed that necrosis in salivary gland neoplasms is not necessarily a sign of malignant transformation [6].

The value of tumor markers in the diagnosis of salivary gland tumors is rather limited. This subject will thus only be briefly discussed in the histological descriptions of the several neoplasms, whereappropriate. The ultrastructural aspects of the various salivary gland neoplasms will not be discussed in detail either, since there is rarely any need for electron microscopy examination for making a diagnosis of a salivary gland neoplasm.

In general, histological typing of salivary tumors can be quite difficult, not only with regard to the typing within the benign or the malignant categories, but also with regard to the benign or malignant nature of the neoplasm [192, 197, 199]. The use of fresh-frozen sections during surgery may thus be hazardous [89, 119, 162].

Table 5.2. Histological classification of epithelial salivary gland tumours [168]

1	**Adenomas**
1.1	Pleomorphic adenoma
1.2	Myoepithelioma (myoepithelial adenoma)
1.3	Basal cell adenoma
1.4	Warthin tumor (adenolymphoma)
1.5	Oncocytoma (oncocytic adenoma)
1.6	Canalicular adenoma
1.7	Sebaceous adenoma
1.8	Ductal papilloma
1.9	Cystadenoma
2	**Carcinomas**
2.1	Acinic cell carcinoma
2.2	Mucoepidermoid carcinoma
2.3	Adenoid cystic carcinoma
2.4	Polymorphous low-grade adenocarcinoma (terminal duct adenocarcinoma)
2.5	Epithelial–myoepithelial carcinoma
2.6	Basal cell adenocarcinoma
2.7	Sebaceous carcinoma
2.8	Papillary cystadenocarcinoma
2.9	Mucinous adenocarcinoma
2.10	Oncocytic carcinoma
2.11	Salivary duct carcinoma
2.12	Adenocarcinoma
2.13	Malignant myoepithelioma (myoepithelial carcinoma)
2.14	Carcinoma in pleomorphic adenoma (malignant mixed tumor)
2.15	Squamous cell carcinoma
2.16	Small cell carcinoma
2.17	Undifferentiated carcinoma
2.18	Other carcinomas

5.8.1 Adenomas

5.8.1.1 Pleomorphic Adenoma

A pleomorphic adenoma is a tumor of variable capsulation characterized microscopically by architectural rather than cellular pleomorphisms. Epithelial and modified myoepithelial elements intermingle with tissue of mucoid, myxoid, or chondroid appearance. The epithelial and myoepithelial component form ducts, strands, sheets, or structures resembling a swarm of bees. Squamous metaplasia is found in about 25% of pleomorphic adenomas (Figs. 5.16, 5.17) [168].

Pleomorphic adenomas are usually solitary and well-circumscribed, except in cases of local recurrence. In rare instances, capsular invasion or satellite nodules may be observed.

In general, diagnosis of a pleomorphic adenoma is not difficult to make histologically, although a chordoma may be misinterpreted as a pleomorphic adenoma [132]. Occasionally, clear cells are observed in pleomorphic adenomas. Squamous metaplasia can also be present. Several types of crystalloids have been reported to occur in pleomorphic adenomas [103, 204]. Such crystalloids apparently may give rise to the formation of granulomas [188]. Apart from tissue of mucoid, myxoid, or chondroid appearance, foci of osteoid tissue and lipometaplasia may be observed [151].

Attempts have been made to subclassify pleomorphic adenomas on the basis of immunohistochemical analysis [11] or morphology. However, in general such subtyping has little or no clinical relevance.

There may be marked cellularity, and cellular pleomorphism and mitotic activity may occasionally be observed [45]. In a small percentage of pleomorphic adenomas, malignant transformation takes place.

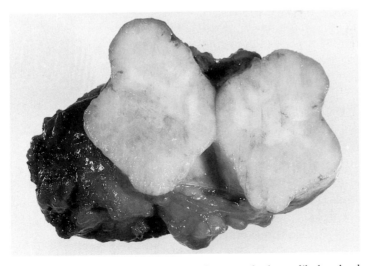

Fig. 5.16. Cut surface of pleomorphic adenoma of submandibular gland

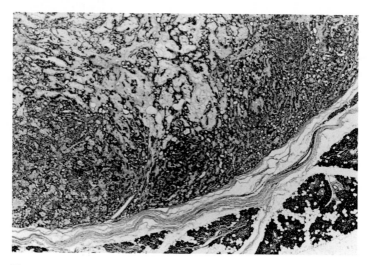

Fig. 5.17. Low-power view of pleomorphic adenoma of parotid gland. Note the demarcation between the neoplastic tissue and the surrounding parotid gland tissue at the bottom

This so-called carcinoma in pleomorphic adenoma will be discussed later (see Sect. 5.8.2.14). Apparently, the expression of proliferating cell nuclear antigen cannot be used in the prediction of malignant transformation potential [212].

A few cases have been reported of metastatic pleomorphic adenomas in which both the primary and the metastatic lesion failed to show any features of malignancy [206].

5.8.1.2 Myoepithelioma (Myoepithelial Adenoma)

A myoepithelioma is a rare tumor of myoepithelial cells; several growth patterns occur, i.e., solid, myxoid, and reticular [168].

Many studies have dealt with the identification of myoepithelial cells in human salivary glands [55]. A myoepithelial cell-specific monoclonal antikeratin is not yet available, although immunohistochemistry with an antibody to smooth muscle actin on frozen tissue seems to be quite helpful. The demonstration of actin and S-100 protein is also valuable in this respect. It has also been suggested that vimentin can be used to define the participation and distribution of myoepithelial cells [9]. Glial acidic fibrillary protein may be one of the most reliable markers for myoepithelioma [52].

Myoepithelial cells sometimes have a homogeneous eosinophilic cytoplasm and have been called hyaline or plasmacytoid cells. Some authors have questioned the myoepithelial cell origin of the plasmacytoid cells [76].

In the past, the myoepithelioma has been considered a subtype of pleomorphic adenoma. The distinction is perhaps important, because the myoepithelioma is said to be characterized by more aggressive growth than the pleomorphic adenoma and occasionally by transformation to malignancy (see Sect. 5.8.2.13), thus requiring different treatment; some authors have questioned this view [153]. The nuclear DNA content might correlate with prognosis [108].

5.8.1.3 Basal Cell Adenoma

A basal cell adenoma is a tumor of isomorphic basaloid cells with a prominent basal cell layer, a distinct basement membrane-like structure, and no mucoid stromal component as in pleomorphic adenomas. Four cellular patterns occur: solid, trabecular, tubular, and membranous (dermal anlage type) [168].

The membranous variant of basal cell adenoma of the salivary glands may be associated with dermal cylindromas (trichoepitheliomas) of the skin of the head, supporting the hypothesis of a common histogenesis of the skin and salivary gland tumors.

Basal cell adenomas comprise 1%–2% of all salivary gland tumors, with an age peak in the seventh decade of life. The main locations are the parotid gland and the minor salivary glands of the upper lip. In the latter location, multifocal presentation is not uncommon (Fig. 5.18). A few cases have been reported that apparently developed from ectopic salivary tissue in lymph nodes [128].

5.8.1.4 Warthin Tumor (Adenolymphoma)

The Warthin tumor is a tumor composed of glandular and often cystic structures, sometimes with a papillary cystic arrangement,

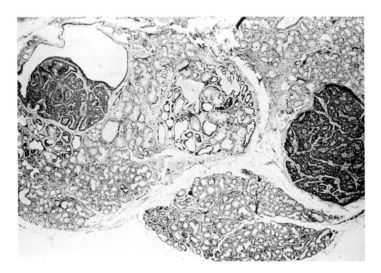

Fig. 5.18. Multifocal presentation of basal cell adenoma of upper lip

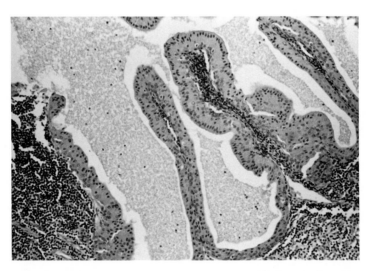

Fig. 5.19. Characteristic papillary projections in cystic lumen of Warthin tumor

lined by characteristic eosinophilic epithelium. The stroma contains a variable amount of lymphoid tissue with follicles (Fig. 5.19) [168].

The Warthin tumor probably arises from salivary gland epithelium entrapped in a lymph node. It is striking that hardly any other types of salivary gland tumors arise from epithelium that has been entrapped in lymph nodes. In predisposed individuals, Epstein-Barr virus (EBV) in latent sites of infection, such as the parotid gland, might infect ductal epithelial cells, followed by a polyclonal B cell response [78].

The Warthin tumor is more or less limited to the parotid glands [67]. Few cases of extraparotid occurrence of Warthin tumor have been reported [2, 64, 200]. Approximately 10% of all parotid gland neoplasms fall into this category. However, in a series of 83 tumors of the parotid glands reported from Malawi, not a single Warthin tumor was observed [190].

Bilateral occurrence, either synchronous or metachronous, is not uncommon. In rare cases, multifocality within one parotid gland may be encountered. The combination of a Warthin tumor and another salivary gland neoplasm, usually a pleomorphic adenoma, may also be seen [121].

In contrast to most other salivary gland neoplasms, the Warthin tumor results almost invariably in a hot spot on the scintigram. The sialogram shows a benign neoplasm.

There is a strong preference for occurrence in males, usually after the sixth decade. However, in a series of 42 patients in the United States, an equal distribution between men and women was observed [145].

Some exceptional cases of malignancy have been reported, either of the epithelial [146, 154] or the lymphocytic component [39, 138]. A rare case of a Warthin tumor and a coexistent Hodgkin's lymphoma has been reported [16].

5.8.1.5 Oncocytoma (Oncocytic Adenoma)

An oncocytoma is a rare tumor composed of a well-demarcated mass of polyhedral eosinophilic cells with small, dark nuclei. It has a solid, trabecular, or tubular pattern and frequently contains both light and dark cells (Fig. 5.20) [168].

An oncocytoma probably arises from the intercalated duct reserve cell. From a histopathologic viewpoint, the distinction between oncocytosis, oncocytic hyperplasia, and a neoplasm of oncycytes is somewhat difficult to define [157]. When the oncocytes follow the

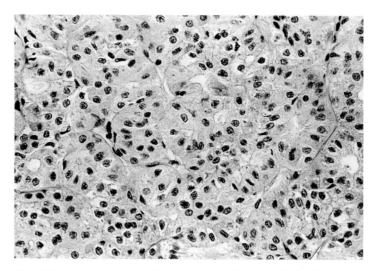

Fig. 5.20. Low-power view of oncocytoma of the parotid gland

preexisting architecture of the gland, the term *oncocytosis* is used. When there is multifocality, the term *multifocal oncocytic adenomatous hyperplasia* is used. In the case of distinct proliferation of oncocytes, the term *oncocytoma* should be used. A few cases of oncocytic carcinomas have been reported (see Sect. 5.8.2.10).

The intensely eosinophylic granular cytoplasm is due to large numbers of mitochondria. Cytoplasmic staining of mitochondria with phosphotungstic acid-hematoxylin (PTAH) can be helpful for the diagnosis of oncocytes. A number of so-called clear cell oncocytomas have been reported [60]. In some cases of oncocytoma, the presence of psammoma bodies has been observed [69].

There is very little stroma, and although lymphocytes may occasionally be present, lymphoid follicles are rarely seen, in contrast to the Warthin tumor.

Oncocytoma is a rare tumor that predominantly occurs in the parotid gland of older adults [33]. Intraoral occurrence is very uncommon. The same holds true for occurrence in the submandibular gland [136].

Like the Warthin tumor, the oncocytoma produces a hot spot on the scintigram.

5.8.1.6 Canalicular Adenoma

A canalicular adenoma is an adenoma of columnar epithelial cells arranged in anastomosing bilayered strands that form a beading pattern. The stroma is loose, highly vascular, and not fibrous as in basal cell adenomas [168].

In 90% of cases, the canalicular adenoma is located in the upper lip and usually occurs in patients over 50 years of age. Multiple occurrence is sometimes referred to as adenomatosis [113].

Canalicular adenomas seem to be derived from cells of excretory ducts [137].

5.8.1.7 Sebaceous Adenoma

A sebaceous adenoma is a rare tumor consisting of irregular nests of sebaceous cells without cellular atypia. The tumor is typically well circumscribed and cystic [168].

Sebaceous lymphadenoma is a rare, but distinctive variant of sebaceous adenoma.

5.8.1.8 Ductal Papilloma

Ductal papillomas occur almost exclusively in the minor salivary glands [75]. The WHO classification recognizes three subtypes [168]:

1. Inverted ductal papilloma [44]
2. Intraductal papilloma [106]
3. Sialadenoma papilliferum [46, 202]

Histologically, inverted ductal papillomas resemble the inverted papilloma of the nose and paranasal sinuses, but they are completely benign and are not associated with malignant change [97].

5.8.1.9 Cystadenoma

Papillary Cystadenoma. A papillary cystadenoma is a tumor that closely resembles the Warthin tumor but without the lymphoid elements [168]. Most cases have been described in the larynx; occurrence in the salivary glands is rare.

Mucinous Cystadenoma. A mucinous cystadenoma is a circumscribed tumor with cystic spaces lined by mucus-producing cells or goblet cells, but no cellular atypia or invasive growth [168]. Great care is needed to differentiate this tumor from its more common malignant counterpart, mucinous adenocarcinoma (see Sect. 5.8.2.9). The diagnosis is based on the encapsulation of the tumor and absence of cellular atypia.

5.8.2 Carcinomas

5.8.2.1 Acinic Cell Carcinoma

An acinic cell carcinoma is a malignant epithelial neoplasm that demonstrates some cytological differentiation toward acinar cells (Fig. 5.21) [168].

The acinic cell carcinoma is usually well circumscribed, but local invasive growth may also be encountered. Pleomorphism or mitotic

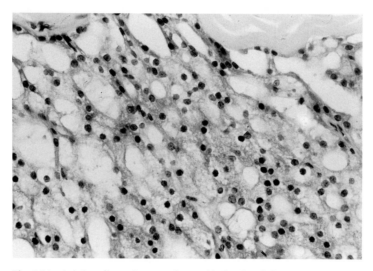

Fig. 5.21. Acinic cell carcinoma of parotid gland, solid type

activity is quite uncommon. In some instances, abundant lymphoid tissue is present in the stroma. Four growth patterns may occur [122]:

1. Solid parenchymatous mass composed of sheets of tumor cells
2. Microcystic configuration with numerous small cystic spaces
3. Papillary cystic configuration with papillae in the spaces
4. Follicular pattern resembling that of thyroid follicles

There is probably only limited value in histological grading of an acinic cell carcinoma, as metastases may occur regardless of the histological type [22, 47, 61]. The same holds true for the prognostic relevance of DNA flow cytometry and nucleolar organizer regions [95, 191].

When the tumor cells appear as clear cells, the possibility of a clear cell variant of a mucoepidermoid carcinoma and metastatic growth of a renal cell carcinoma or a thyroid carcinoma should be considered [156]. The clear cells in acinic cell carcinoma are usually periodic acid-Schiff (PAS) positive and diastase resistant. However, clear cells in salivary gland tissue may also be an artifact caused by prolonged formalin fixation [65].

Acinic cell carcinomas are much more common in the parotid gland than in the submandibular gland, the minor salivary gland taking an intermediate position in this respect. Intraosseous occurrence in the mandible or the maxilla is extremely rare. An exceptional case of an acinic cell carcinoma arising in a parotid lymph node has been reported [144].

5.8.2.2 Mucoepidermoid Carcinoma

A mucoepidermoid carcinoma is a tumor characterized by the presence of squamous cells, mucus-producing cells, and cells of intermediate type (Fig. 5.22) [168].

The proportion of the different tumor cells may vary considerably. Interestingly, keratin pearl formation is uncommon in mucoepidermoid carcinoma. Some of the epidermoid cells may undergo hydropic degeneration, resulting in so-called clear cells. The clear cells are often mucin negative, but may contain glycogen, typically in the form of droplets rather than granules [65]. In rare cases, melanin pigment may be encountered in a mucoepidermoid carcinoma [15].

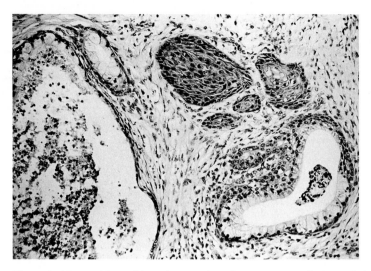

Fig. 5.22. Mucoepidermoid carcinoma. Note the mucous-producing cells in the cyst-like spaces and the epidermoid islands

Quite often, the tumor is cystic and fairly well circumscribed. However, local invasive growth may occur. Histological grading of a mucoepidermoid carcinoma is usually based on the proportion of epidermoid and mucous cells, cellular differentiation, mitotic activity, and the presence or absence of local invasiveness. Thus a well-differentiated (low-grade), a moderately differentiated (intermediate-grade), and a poorly differentiated (high-grade) mucoepidermoid carcinoma can be recognized [29]. In a study of 143 intraoral cases, the histopathologic features that indicated high-grade behavior were an intracystic component of less than 20%, four or more mitotic figures per ten high-power fields, neural invasion, necrosis, and cellular anaplasia [14]. In another study, patients with diploid tumors were shown to do better than those with aneuploid ones; furthermore, proliferative activity was found to be a prognostic factor [93, 99]. The argyrophilic nucleolar organizer region(AgNOR) may have a prognostic significance [43].

It should be realized that any mucoepidermoid carcinoma may metastasize, whatever its histological grade of differentiation.

The mucoepidermoid carcinoma is one of the rare salivary gland neoplasms that may be encountered centrally in the jaw bones, especially in the mandible [68]. A rare case of primary muco-epidermoid carcinoma in an intraparotid lymph node has been reported [189].

5.8.2.3 Adenoid Cystic Carcinoma

ACC is an infiltrative malignant tumor having various histological features with three growth patterns, glandular (cribriform), tubular, or solid. The tumor cells are of two types, duct-lining cells and cells of the myoepithelial type. Perineural or perivascular spread without stromal reaction is very characteristic. All structural types of ACC can be associated in the same tumor (Fig. 5.23) [168].

ACC may be well circumscribed in some areas, but usually shows distinct areas of infiltration. The perineural and endoneural extension of the tumor cells is well known and influences the prognosis [195]. Endoneural spread should not be confused with the exceptional finding of benign glandular inclusions that have been reported to occur in parotid nerves [51]. Invasion of the blood vessels is also quite common, whereas spread to the cervical lymph nodes is rare.

ACC is made up of cells of the myoepithelial type and of cells similar to those that line normal salivary ducts. These two cell types may grow in different patterns, such as the glandular (cribriform), the tubular, and the solid (basaloid) type. The pseudocysts in ACC contain mucoid material which strongly reacts with alcian blue. Squamous metaplasia rarely occurs in ACC [198].

Occasionally, it may be difficult to distinguish with certainty between an ACC and a cellular pleomorphic adenoma, a basal cell adenoma, a basal cell adenocarcinoma (BCAC), and a polymorphous low-grade adenocarcinoma. In intraoral ACC, the possibility of a basaloid squamous cell carcinoma should also be considered.

ACC is relatively common in the intraoral salivary glands. Even intraosseous occurrence in the mandible can be observed, in some cases as a result of secondary invasion. When occurring in the palatal or maxillary bone, it is sometimes difficult to assess whether the tumor has originated from an intraoral site or from the nasal cavity or the maxillary sinus. Minimal bone resorption may be observed on radiographs even when the tumor cells have extensively infiltrated the bone marrow spaces [184].

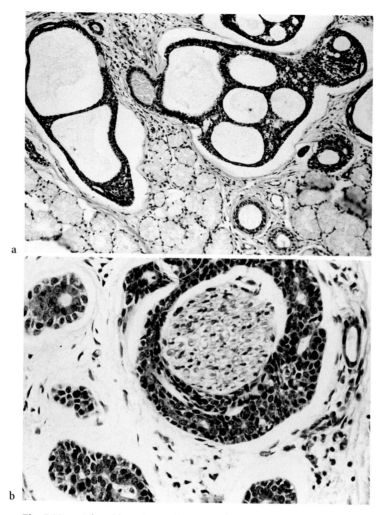

Fig. 5.23. a Adenoid cystic carcinoma, cribriform type, infiltrating normal mucous glands. **b** Perineural spread is a common feature

It has been claimed that the biological behavior of the adenoid cystic carcinoma correlates with the histological subtypes, the solid type having the worst prognosis, the tubular type the best, and the glandular type an intermediate position [115, 185]. The volume-weighted mean volume of tumor nuclei appears to be an indicator of short-term treatment failure [211]. DNA aneuploidy and S-phase fractions are also considered to be potential prognostic factors, indicating that DNA flow cytometry may assist in the biological characterization of ACC [18, 77, 96, 129]. Counts of nucleolar organizer regions do not seem to be a prognostic factor [74].

5.8.2.4 Polymorphous Low-Grade Adenocarcinoma (Terminal Duct Adenocarcinoma)

A polymorphous low-grade adenocarcinoma (terminal duct adenocarcinoma) is a malignant epithelial tumor characterized by cytological uniformity, morphological diversity, and a low metastatic potential [168].

Macroscopically, the tumor may appear to be circumscribed, but microscopically invasion and lack of encapsulation may be observed. The cells are often pale, and mitoses are rare.

The WHO classification recognizes four different patterns:

1. Lobular
2. Papillary or papillary–cystic
3. Cribriform, sometimes closely resembling ACC
4. Trabecular

Furthermore, it has been described that the cells may form whorls around nerves and blood vessels, not to be confused with ACC.

Polymorphous low-grade adenocarcinoma has been claimed to show a different staining pattern of epithelial membrane antigen (EMA) and carcinoembryonic antigen (CEA) compared to the staining pattern in ACC [84]. According to others, however, the immunohistochemical reactions are not sufficiently dissimilar to be of practical value [175].

Polymorphous low-grade adenocarcinomas are almost exclusively found in the oral cavity, especially in the palate [48, 163, 194]. There is a marked predilection for occurrence in women and a mean age of presentation in the sixth decade [127]. The prognosis is favorable.

5.8.2.5 Epithelial–Myoepithelial Carcinoma

An epithelial–myoepithelial carcinoma is a tumor composed of variable proportions of two cell types which typically form duct-like structures. There is an inner layer of duct-lining cells and an outer layer of clear cells [168].

The epithelial–myoepithelial carcinoma accounts for approximately 1% of all salivary gland neoplasms [27]. It mainly occurs in the parotid glands in older patients. The outer clear cells stain strongly for glycogen and are positive for S-100 protein, actin, and myosin. Occurrence in minor salivary glands is very rare [91].

Epithelial–myoepithelial carcinoma is associated with a variable prognosis. In a series of 22 patients, 40% died of their disease [73], while in another study of 21 patients with a mean follow-up of 118 months, none died of their disease [94].

5.8.2.6 Basal Cell Adenocarcinoma

Basal Cell Adenocarcinoma (BCAC) is an epithelial neoplasm that has cytological characteristics of basal cell adenoma, but a morphological growth pattern indicative of malignancy [168].

The term BCAC distinguishes this tumor from the basal cell carcinoma of the skin.

Coexistence with dermal cylindroma has been observed in 10% of cases. BCAC is regarded as the malignant counterpart of benign basal cell adenoma. In contrast to basal cell adenoma, two signs of BCAC are important for the diagnosis: (1) frequent mitoses and (2) infiltrative growth, including perineural and intravascular infiltration [133].

BCAC is considered to be of low-grade malignancy, giving rise to metastases in not more than 10% of cases [65]. It occurs predominantly in the parotid glands, and intraoral occurrence is rare [125].

5.8.2.7 Sebaceous Carcinoma

A sebaceous carcinoma is a rare variety of carcinoma composed of sebaceous cells of varying degrees of maturity [168].

Sebaceous lymphadenocarcinoma is a very rare variety of sebaceous carcinoma. It is the malignant counterpart of sebaceous lymphadenoma. It seems likely that sebaceous carcinoma originates from pluripotential duct cells which can differentiate into sebaceous, ductal, and mucous cells [187].

5.8.2.8 Papillary Cystadenocarcinoma

A papillary cystadenocarcinoma is a malignant tumor characterized by cysts and papillary endocystic projections [168].

The term papillary cystadenocarcinoma is applied to adenocarcinomas in which only papillary structures are present. Papillary adenocarcinoma is considered to be a low-grade carcinoma, although some authors claim that it shows a more aggressive biological behavior compared with other low-grade adenocarcinomas in this region [147]. Indeed, the term "papillary low-grade adenocarcinoma" should no longer be used [177].

In the differential diagnosis, the possibility of a metastasis of papillary thyroid carcinoma should be taken into account.

5.8.2.9 Mucinous Adenocarcinoma

A mucinous adenocarcinoma is a rare tumor characterized by abundant mucus production [168].

The mucus should occupy more than 50% of the tumor, and epidermoid or intermediate cells should not be present. Very few cases have been reported [155].

5.8.2.10 Oncocytic Carcinoma

An oncocytic carcinoma is a very rare tumor composed of malignant oncocytic cells [168].

Cellular and nuclear pleomorphism may be present, but is not sufficient to confirm malignancy. Additional criteria for malignancy are local infiltration, perineural or intravascular invasion, and lymph node or distant metastasis. Oncocytic carcinoma is often, but not always associated with a poor prognosis [33, 88].

5.8.2.11 Salivary Duct Carcinoma

A salivary duct carcinoma (SDC) is an epithelial tumor of high malignancy with formation of relatively large cell aggregates resembling distended salivary ducts. The neoplastic epithelium presents a combination of cribriform, looping ("Roman bridging"), and solid growth patterns, often with central necrosis both in the primary lesions and the lymph node metastases [168].

The characteristic features of SDC include papillary and cribriform patterns, together with so-called comedo necrosis. SDC arise almost exclusively in the major salivary glands, especially in the parotid glands, and are three times more common in men than in women [19]. In a study of 15 SDC patients, three preexisting pleomorphic adenomas were identified [57].

A diagnosis of SDC carries a poor prognosis [3, 8, 49, 148, 174].

5.8.2.12 Adenocarcinoma

An adenocarcinoma is a carcinoma with glandular, ductal, or secretory differentiation that does not fit into the other categories of carcinoma [168].

The histological architecture and cellular features may be extremely variable. If no further subtyping can be given, the designation NOS ("not otherwise specified") is applied. These are the least common of the salivary carcinomas and display a cytoarchitecture ranging from a well-differentiated, low-grade appearance to high-grade, invasive lesions [26].

5.8.2.13 Malignant Myoepithelioma (Myoepithelial Carcinoma)

A malignant myoepithelioma (myoepithelial carcinoma) is a rare malignant epithelial tumor composed of atypical myoepithelial cells with increased mitotic activity and aggressive growth [168].

Only a few cases of malignant myoepitheliomas have been reported [59].

5.8.2.14 Carcinoma in Pleomorphic Adenoma
(Malignant Mixed Tumor)

Carcinomas in pleomorphic adenoma (malignant mixed tumors) are tumors which show definitive evidence of malignancy, such as cytological and histological characteristics of anaplasia, abnormal mitoses, progressive course, and infiltrative growth, and in which evidence of pleomorphic adenoma can still be found [168].

Malignant change in a pleomorphic adenoma probably occurs in about 2% of all such tumors, especially in those of long duration. In some series, this event seems more likely to occur in men. The histology of the malignant part may assume the features of several of the malignant salivary neoplasms that have been discussed previously and may even show a mixed pattern. It is rare to observe the features of ACC in these circumstances.

The WHO has recommended that the use of the term "carcinoma in pleomorphic adenoma" be limited to those cases in which areas of pleomorphic adenoma can still be identified in addition to malignant

Table 5.3. Nomenclature for benign and malignant mixed (pleomorphic) tumors [54]

Class	Criteria
Pleomorphic adenoma (PA)	Benign epithelial and mesenchymal components
Metastasizing pleomorphic adenoma	Histologically benign, but biologically malignant tumor
Pleomorphic carcinoma – Noninvasive (intracapsular) – Invading normal salivary gland	De novo malignant tumor with the histological growth pattern and myxoid stroma seen in PA; no historic or evidence for a preexisting PA
Carcinoma ex pleomorphic adenoma – Noninvasive (intracapsular) – Invasive	The malignant component (squamous, adenocarcinoma, or undifferentiated carcinoma) lacks the histological growth pattern and myxoid stroma seen in PA, but preexisting benign epithelial and mesenchymal elements typical of a PA are present
True malignant mixed tumor (carcinosarcoma)	Malignant epithelial and mesenchymal components with or without preexisting PA

tissue. Dardick et al. [54] proposed a nomenclature for benign and malignant mixed (pleomorphic) tumors, outlined in Table 5.3, that differs slightly from the WHO recommendations.

The exceptional event of a histologically benign pleomorphic adenoma that produces a metastatic lesion has been previously mentioned (see Sect. 5.8.1.1). Some authors recognize a so-called *true* malignant mixed tumor or carcinosarcoma of the salivary glands in which malignant features are encountered both in the epithelial part and the stromal part [31, 82].

5.8.2.15 Squamous Cell Carcinoma

A squamous cell carcinoma is a malignant epithelial tumor with cells forming keratin or having intercellular bridges. Mucus secretion is not present [168].

A pure squamous cell carcinoma of salivary gland origin is fairly rare. In a series of 48 cases, the majority were located in the parotid gland [171]. When dealing with a squamous cell carcinoma in the parotid or submandibular region, the possibility of metastasis rather than a primary tumor should be considered initially.

Aggressive treatment and early detection of a primary squamous cell carcinoma may result in a better prognosis than is commonly associated with these tumors [83].

5.8.2.16 Small Cell Carcinoma

A small cell carcinoma is a malignant tumor similar in histology, behavior, and histochemistry to the small cell carcinoma of the lung [168].

These tumors may resemble oat cell carcinomas of the lung and are often referred to as neuroendocrine small cell carcinomas [104, 165]. The tumor cells are thought to be derived from neural crest cells [87]. There are also non-neuroendocrine small cell carcinomas. In a report by the Armed Forces Institute of Pathology on 12 cases of small cell carcinoma of the major salivary glands, only one true neuroendocrine ('oat cell') carcinoma was observed; most of the other tumors were actually small ductal carcinomas [85]. There is also a report of a small round cell tumor of the parotid region with features of extraskeletal Ewing's sarcoma [214].

5.8.2.17 Undifferentiated Carcinoma

An undifferentiated carcinoma is a malignant tumor of epithelial structure that is too poorly differentiated, i.e., is devoid of any phenotypic expression by light microscopy, to be placed in any of the other groups of carcinoma [168].

The entity of "undifferentiated carcinoma with lymphoid stroma" has been accepted in preference to terms such as malignant lymphoepithelial lesion or lymphoepithelial carcinoma [30, 117]. There is a relatively high incidence in Chinese and Greenlandic Eskimos [92], and there seems to be a consistent and specific association between Epstein-Barr virus and the tumor cells [5].

The single most important clinicopathologic factor influencing the outcome of the disease is size of the primary tumor [102].

5.8.2.18 Other Carcinomas

In the literature, several cases of clear cell tumors or carcinomas, with or without hyalinization, have been published, apparently representing tumors of low malignant potential [23, 141, 176]. In general, however, the use of the term "clear cell" salivary gland tumor is discouraged in the revised WHO classification. Instead, such tumors should be classified as subtypes of entities such as mucoepidermoid carcinoma and acinic cell carcinoma.

A rare case of carcinoma of the parotid gland has been reported with osteoclast-like giant cells [17], and a few cases of giant cell tumors in the parotid gland have been reported in the literature [63].

5.9 Treatment and Prognosis

5.9.1 General Comments

In general, treatment of a salivary gland neoplasm consists of surgical removal. It is beyond the scope of this chapter to deal with the various surgical aspects in much detail. The type of surgical modality employed is usually influenced to some extent by the availability of postoperative radiotherapy. For instance, when dealing with a malignant neoplasm of the parotid gland and an intact facial nerve, most surgeons prefer to perform a fairly conservative surgical parotidectomy, leaving the facial nerve intact. Such a procedure is then followed by a full course of radiotherapy. In high-grade tumors of the major salivary glands, elective treatment of the neck should be considered [10]. Since lymph nodes are present in the deep lobe of the gland, superficial parotidectomy alone does not appear to be adequate when combined with a radical neck dissection [80]. It is also beyond the scope of this text to discuss the aggressive surgical approach in the case of recurrent pleomorphic adenoma of the parotid gland [159].

When dealing with a salivary gland neoplasm of the submandibular gland, most surgeons prefer to perform a supraomohyoid neck dissection [205]. This method is also preferred when dealing with a neoplasm of the floor of the mouth.

In palatal neoplasms, the underlying bone should be included in the specimen when dealing with a malignant type, even in the absence of positive findings on preoperative radiographs or CT scans. Especially when dealing with an ACC in this location, the surgical margins are often positive. Such a deceptive finding can hardly be avoided if fresh-frozen sections are used during the surgical procedure, partly because of the shape and size of the specimen and partly because of the difficulties involved in preparing fresh-frozen sections from bony margins.

5.9.2 Role of Radiotherapy

Primary radiotherapy is generally not used for the treatment of malignant salivary gland neoplasms, with the possible exception of neutron radiotherapy in ACC [38]. Nevertheless, some encouraging reports have been published, e.g., in the treatment of ACC [100]. There is, however, a place for postoperative radiotherapy, especially after surgical removal of a malignant neoplasm in which microscopic rests are likely to be left behind. In many centers, postoperative radiotherapy is routinely used after surgical removal of a malignant salivary gland neoplasm, irrespective of the results of the histological examination of the surgical margins [81, 116, 173, 179, 201]. Postoperative radiotherapy should also be used in cases of nerve involvement [209]. A few cases of combined postoperative radiotherapy and hyperthermia in ACC have been reported [20].

In incomplete removal of a pleomorphic adenoma, recurrences are the rule, becoming manifest as multiple foci many years after the primary surgical treatment. Recurrences are apparently more common in patients who are under 30 years of age at initial presentation [134]. When located in the parotid gland, a recurrence may be extremely difficult to handle without damaging branches of the facial nerve. Thus postoperative irradiation should be considered when there has been tumor spill in the surgical field during the removal of a pleomorphic adenoma of the parotid gland.

5.9.3 Role of Chemotherapy

The role of chemotherapy in the treatment of malignant salivary gland neoplasms is still controversial. A number of encouraging results have been reported [112, 124], while others have reported poor results, not least in cases of advanced malignant salivary gland tumors [90, 109].

5.9.4 Prognosis

The prognosis for patients with malignant salivary gland neoplasms varies with the histological type of the tumor, its size, and its specific location. The relatively indolent course of some histological types of malignant salivary gland tumors might be associated with the preservation of the nonmutated p53 gene in most of these tumors [178]. In another paper, it has been suggested that the p53 tumor suppressor gene is involved in salivary gland carcinogenesis; its oncoprotein expression seems to be an independent indicator of clinical aggressiveness in patients with parotid gland carcinoma [79, 123]. Progesterone receptor expression may be of possible prognostic and therapeutic value in some cases of ACC [172]. The AgNOR count might be a useful prognostic indicator in ACC [196].

Local cure can often be achieved by a combination of aggressive surgery and postoperative radiotherapy, especially in patients with ACC [50, 140]. However, metastatic spread is not uncommon. Such metastatic spread is often delayed beyond the traditional 5-year surveillance period. Clinical stage and persistence of tumor cells are likely to be more important than histological grade for metastasis, and hematogenous metastasis is more frequent than lymphatic spread [24]. In a series of 110 patients with a malignant parotid tumor, facial nerve palsy was an indicator of an extremely poor prognosis [158].

In a few studies of patients with malignant salivary gland tumors, the location of these tumors (minor salivary glands, submandibular gland, parotid gland) had no distinct influence on their prognosis; the most favorable prognosis was found for tubular ACC, well-differentiated acinic cell carcinoma, and low-grade mucoepidermoid carcinomas; the prognosis for solid and glandular (cribriform) ACC, poorly differentiated acinic cell carcinomas, and the salivary duct carcinomas was less favorable, followed by adenocarcinomas, poorly differentiated mucoepidermoid carcinomas, and squamous cell carcinomas; the least favorable prognosis was found in carcinomas ex pleomorphic adenoma and undifferentiated carcinoma [7, 110]. In another study of carcinomas in the major salivary glands, the clinical stage was the most important prognostic variable [181].

In a review of the literature, the 5-year survival rate in patients with ACC was approximately 60%, while the 10-year survival rate was about 40% [114]. In a study of 46 patients with mucoepidermoid carcinoma, the clinical staging and histological grading were shown to be the most important factors influencing survival [149].

References

1. Abbey LM, Schwab BH, Landau GC, et al. Incidence of second primary breast cancer among patients with a first primary salivary gland tumor. Cancer 1984; 54: 1439–1442.
2. Adibfar A, Mintz SM. Papillary cystadenoma lymphomatosum of the upper lip: Report of case. J Oral Maxillofac Surg 1994; 52: 183–185.
3. Afzelius L-E, Cameron WR, Svensson C. Salivary duct carcinoma – a clinicopathologic study of 12 cases. Head & Neck Surgery 1987; 9: 151–156.

4. Akker van den HP. Diagnostic imaging in salivary gland disease. Oral Surg Oral Med Oral Pathol 1988; 66: 625–637.

5. Albeck H, Bentzen J, Ockelmann HH, et al. Familial clusters of nasopharyngeal carcinoma and salivary gland carcinomas in Greenland natives. Cancer 1993; 2: 196–200.

6. Allen CM, Damm D, Neville B, et al. Necrosis in benign salivary gland neoplasms. Not necessarily a sign of malignant transformation. Oral Surg Oral Med Oral Pathol 1994; 78: 455–461.

7. Andersen LJ, Hamilton Therkildsen M, Ockelmann HH, et al. Malignant epithelial tumors in the minor salivary glands, the submandibular gland, and the sublingual gland. Prognostic factors and treatment results. Cancer 1991; 68: 2431–2437.

8. Anderson C, Muller R, Piorkowski R, et al. Intraductal carcinoma of major salivary gland. Cancer 1992; 69: 609–614.

9. Araujo de VC, Carvalho YR, Araujo de NS. Actin versus vimentin in myoepithelial cells of salivary gland tumors. A comparative study. Oral Surg Oral Med Oral Pathol 1994; 77: 387–391.

10. Armstrong JG, Harrison LB, Thaler HT, et al. The indications for elective treatment of the neck in cancer of the major salivary glands. Cancer 1992; 69: 615–619.

11. Aroni K, Fotiou, Liossi A, et al. Immunohistochemical study of four histologic types of parotid gland pleomorphic adenoma. J Oral Pathol Med 1991; 20: 37–40.

12. Auclair PL, Langloss JM, Weiss SW, et al. Sarcomas and sarcomatoid neoplasms of the major salivary gland regions. A clinicopathologic and immunohistochemical study of 67 cases and review of the literature. Cancer 1986; 58: 1305–1315.

13. Auclair PL. Tumor-associated lymphoid proliferation in the parotid gland. A potential diagnostic pitfall. Oral Surg Oral Med Oral Pathol 1994; 77: 19–26.

14. Auclair PL, Goode RK, Ellis GL. Mucoepidermoid carcinoma of intraoral salivary glands. Evaluation and application of grading criteria in 143 cases. Cancer 1992; 69: 2021–2030.

15. Aufdemorte TB, Sickels van JE, Glass BJ. Melanin pigmentation in a mucoepidermoid tumor of a minor salivary gland. J Oral Maxillofac Surg 1985; 43: 876–879.

16. Badve S, Evans G, Madyy S, et al. A case of Warthin's tumour with coexistent Hodgkin's disease. Histopathology 1993; 22: 280–281.

17. Balogh K, Wolbarsht RL, Federman M, et al. Carcinoma of the parotid gland with osteoclastlike giant cells. Arch Pathol Lab Med 1985; 109: 756–761.

18. Bang G, Donath K, Thoresen S, et al. DNA flow cytometry of reclassified subtypes of malignant salivary gland tumors. J Oral Pathol Med 1994; 23: 291–297.

19. Barnes L, Rao U, Krause J, et al. Salivary duct carcinoma. Part I. A clinicopathologic evaluation and DNA image analysis of 13 cases with review of the literature. Oral Surg Oral Med Oral Pathol 1994; 78: 64–73.

20. Barnett TA, Kapp DS, Goffinet DR. Adenoid cystic carcinoma of the salivary glands. Management of recurrent, advanced, or persistent disease with hyperthermia and radiation therapy. Cancer 1990; 65: 2648–2656.

21. Barsotti JB, Westesson P-L, Coniglio JU. Superiority of magnetic resonance over computed tomography for imaging parotid tumor. Ann Otol Rhinol Laryngol 1994; 103: 737–740.

22. Batsakis JG, Luna MA, El-Naggar AK. Histopathologic grading of salivary gland neoplasms. II: Acinic cell carcinomas. Ann Otol Rhinol Laryngol 1990; 99: 929–933.

23. Batsakis JG, El-Naggar AK, Luna MA. Hyalinizing clear cell carcinoma of salivary origin. Ann Otol Rhinol Laryngol 1994; 103: 746–748.

24. Batsakis JG. Metastatic patterns of salivary gland neoplasms. Ann Otol Rhinol Laryngol 1982; 91: 465–466.

25. Batsakis JG, Bautina E. Metastases to major salivary glands. Ann Otol Rhinol Laryngol 1990; 99: 501–503.

26. Batsakis JG, El-Naggar AK, Luna MA. "Adenocarcinoma, not otherwise specified": a diminishing group of salivary carcinomas. Ann Otol Rhinol Laryngol 1992; 101: 102–104.

27. Batsakis JG, El-Naggar AK, Luna MA. Epithelial-myoepithelial carcinoma of salivary glands. Ann Otol Rhinol Laryngol 1992; 101: 540–542.

28. Batsakis JG, Frankenthaler R. Embryoma (sialoblastoma) of salivary glands. Ann Otol Rhinol Laryngol 1992; 101: 958–960.

29. Batsakis JG, Luna MA. Histopathologic grading of salivary gland neoplasms: I. Mucoepidermoid carcinomas. Ann Otol Rhinol Laryngol 1990; 99: 835–838.

30. Batsakis JG, Luna MA. Undifferentiated carcinomas of salivary glands. Ann Otol Rhinol Laryngol 1991; 100: 82–84.

31. Bleiweiss IJ, Huvos AW, Lara J, et al. Carcinosarcoma of the submandibular salivary gland. Immunohistochemical findings. Cancer 1992; 69: 2031–2035.

32. Bradley MJ. Ultrasonography in the investigation of salivary gland disease. Dentomaxillofac Radiol 1993; 22: 115–119.

33. Brandwein MS, Huvos AG. Oncocytic tumors of major salivary glands. A study of 68 cases with follow-up of 44 patients. Am J Surg Pathol 1991; 15: 514–528.

34. Brannon RB, Houston GD, Wampler HW. Gingival salivary gland choristoma. Oral Surg Oral Med Oral Pathol 1986; 61: 185–188.

35. Breton P, Paulus C, Bancel B, et al. Les tumeurs salivaires intra-mandibulaires. A porpos de 3 observations de tumeurs malignes. Rev Stomatol Chir maxillofac 1990; 91: 266–270.

36. Brookstone MS, Huvos AG. Cetral salivary gland tumors of the maxilla and mandible: A clinicopathologic study of 11 cases with an analysis of the literature. J Oral Maxillofac Surg 1992; 50: 229–236.

37. Bruner JM, Batsakis JG. Salivary neoplasms of the jaw bones with particular reference to central mucoepidermoid carcinomas. Ann Otol Rhinol Laryngol 1991; 100: 954–955.

38. Buchholz TA, Shimotakahara SG, Weymuller EA, et al. Neutron radiotherapy for adenoid cystic carcinoma of the head and neck. Arch Otolaryngol Head Neck Surg 1993; 119: 747–752.

39. Bunker ML, Locker J. Warthin's tumor with malignant lymphoma. DNA analysis of paraffin-embedded tissue. Am J Clin Pathol 1989; 91: 341–344.

40. Byrne MN, Spector JG, Garvin CF, et al. Preoperative assessment of parotid masses: a comparative evaluation of radiologic techniques to histopathologic diagnosis. Laryngoscope 1989; 99: 284–292.

41. Califano L, Zupi A, Giardino C. Accuracy in the diagnosis of parotid tumours. J Carnio-Max-Fac Surg 1992; 20: 354–359.

42. Callender DL, Frankenthaler RA, Luna MA, et al. Salivary gland neoplasms in children. Arch Otolaryngol Head Neck Surg 1992; 118: 472–476.

43. Chomette GP, Auriol MM, Labrousse F, et al. Mucoepidermoid tumors of salivary glands: histoprognostic value of NORs stained with AgNOR technique. J Oral Pathol Med 1991; 20: 130–132.

44. Clark DB, Priddy RW, Swanson AE. Oral inverted ductal papilloma. Oral Surg Oral Med Oral Pathol 1990; 69: 487–490.

45. Clark J, Bailey BMW, Eveson JW. Dysplastic pleomorphic adenoma of the sublingual salivary gland. Br J Oral Maxillofac Surg 1993; 31: 394–395.

46. Cleary KR, Batsakis JG. Sialadenoma papilliferum. Ann Otol Rhinol Laryngol 1990; 99: 756–758.

47. Colmenero C, Patron M, Sierra I. Acinic cell carcinoma of the salivary glands. A review of 20 new cases. J Cranio-Max-Fac Surg 1991; 19: 260–266.

48. Colmenero CM, Patron M, Burgueño M, et al. Polymorphous low-grade adenocarcinoma of the oral cavity: a report of 14 cases. J Oral Maxillofac Surg 1992; 50: 595–600.

49. Colmenero Ruiz C, Patrón Romero M, Martín Pérez M. Salivary duct carcinoma: a report of nine cases. J Oral Maxillofac Surg 1993; 51: 641–646.

50. Coustal B, Diop R, Demaux H, et al. Carcinomes adénoïdes kystiques des glandes salivaires. Intérêt de la radiothérapie post-opératoire. Rev Stomatol Chir maxillofac 1993; 94: 166–169.

51. Cramer SF, Heggeness LM. Benign glandular inclusions in parotid nerve. Am J Clin Pathol 1988; 89: 220–222.

52. Dardick I. Myoepithelioma: definitions and diagnostic criteria. Ultrastruct Pathol 1995; 19: 335–345.

53. Dardick I, Byard RW, Carnegie JA. A review of the proliferative capacity of major salivary glands and the relationship to current concepts of neoplasia in salivary glands. Oral Surg Oral Med Oral Pathol 1990; 69: 53–67.

54. Dardick I, Hardie J, Thomas MJ, et al. Ultrastructural contributions to the study of morphological differentiation in malignant mixed (pleomorphic) tumors of salivary gland. Head & Neck 1989; 11: 5–21.

55. Dardick I, Thomas MJ, van Nostrand AWP. Myoepithelioma – new concepts of histology and classification: a light and electron microscopic study. Ultrastruct Pathol 1989; 13: 187–224.

56. Dehner LP, Valbuena L, Perez-Atayde A, et al. Salivary gland anlage tumor ("Congenital pleomorphic adenoma"). A clinicopathologic, immunohistochemical and ultrastructural study of nine cases. Am J Surg Pathol 1994; 18: 25–36.

57. Delgado R, Vuitch F, Albores-Saavedra J. Salivary duct carcinoma. Cancer 1993; 72: 1503–1512.
58. Dimery IW, Jones LA, Verjan RP, et al. Estrogen receptors in normal salivary gland and salivary gland carcinoma. Arch Otolaryngol Head Neck Surg 1987; 113: 1082–1085.
59. Di Palma S, Pilotti S, Rilke F. Malignant myo-epithelioma of the parotid gland arising in a pleomorphic adenoma. Histopathology 1991; 19: 273–275.
60. Ellis GL. "Clear cell" oncocytoma of salivary gland. Hum Pathol 1988; 19: 862–867.
61. Ellis GL, Corio RL. Acinic cell carcinoma. A clinicopathologic analysis of 294 cases. Cancer 1983; 52: 542–549.
62. El-Naggar AK, Ordóñez NG, Batsakis JG. Parotid gland plasmacytoma with crystalline deposits. Oral Surg Oral Med Oral Pathol 1991; 71: 206–208.
63. Eusebi V, Martin SA, Govoni E, et al. Giant cell tumor of major salivary glands: Report of three cases, one occurring in association with a malignant mixed tumor. Am J Clin Pathol 1984; 81: 666–675.
64. Eveson JW, Cawson RA. Tumours of the minor (oropharyngeal) salivary glands: a demographic study of 336 cases. J Oral Pathol 1985; 14: 500–509.
65. Eveson JW. Troublesome tumours 2: borderline tumours of salivary glands. J Clin Pathol 1992; 45: 369–377.
66. Eveson JW, Cawson RA. Salivary gland tumours. A review of 2410 cases with particular reference to histological types, site, age and sex distribution. J Pathol 1985; 146: 51–58.
67. Eveson JW, Cawson RA. Warthin's tumor (cystadenolymphoma) of salivary glands. A clinicopathologic investigation of 278 cases. Oral Surg Oral Med Oral Pathol 1986; 61: 256–262.
68. Ëzsiás A, Sugar AW, Milling MAP, et al. Central mucoepidermoid carcinoma in a child. J Oral Maxillofac Surg 1994; 52: 512–515.
69. Feiner HD, Goldstein S, Ittman M, et al. Oncocytic adenoma of the parotid gland with psammoma bodies. Arch Pathol Lab Med 1986; 110: 640–644.
70. Fière A, Cartier E, Breton P, et al. Intérêt de la cytoponction à l'aiguille fine dans le diagnostic des tuméfactions des glandes salivaires. Rev Stomatol Chir maxillofac 1990; 91: 291–294.
71. Fischer JR, Abdul-Karim FW, Robinson RA. Intraparotid nodular fasciitis. Arch Pathol Lab Med 1989; 113: 1276–1278.
72. Fonseca I, Martins AG, Soares J. Epithelial salivary gland tumors of children and adolescents in southern Portugal. A clinicopathologic study of twenty-four cases. Oral Surg Oral Med Oral Pathol 1991; 72: 696–701.
73. Fonseca I, Soares J. Epithelial-myoepithelial carcinoma of the salivary glands. A study of 22 cases. Virchows Archiv A Pathol Anat 1993; 422: 389–396.
74. Fonseca I, Soares J. Adenoid cystic carcinoma: a study of nucleolar organizer regions (AgNOR) counts and their relation to prognosis. J Pathology 1993; 169: 255–258.
75. Franklin CD, Ong TK. Ductal papilloma of the minor salivary gland. Histopathology 1991; 19: 180–182.

76. Franquemont DW, Mills SE. Plasmacytoid monomorphic adenoma of salivary glands. Absence of myogenous differentiation and comparison to spindle cell myoepithelioma. Am J Surg Pathol 1993; 17: 146–153.

77. Franzén G, Nordgård S, Boysen M, et al. DNA content in adenoid cystic carcinomas. Head & Neck 1995; 17: 49–55.

78. Gallo O. New insights into the pathogenesis of Warthin's tumour. Oral Oncol, Eur J Cancer 1995; 31B: 211–215.

79. Gallo O, Franchi A, Bianchi S, et al. p53 Oncoprotein expression in parotid gland carcinoma is associated with clinical outcome. Cancer 1995; 75: 2037–2044.

80. Garatea-Crelgo J, Gray-Escoda C, Bermejo B, et al. Morphological study of the parotid lymph nodes. J Cranio-Max-Fac Surg 1993; 21: 207–209.

81. Garden AS, Weber RS, Kian Ang K, et al. Postoperative radiation therapy for malignant tumors of minor salivary glands. Cancer 1994; 73: 2563–2569.

82. Garner SL, Robinson RA, Maves MD, et al. Salivary gland carcinosarcoma: true malignant mixed tumor. Ann Otol Rhinol Laryngol 1989; 98: 611–614.

83. Gaughan RK, Olsen KD, Lewis JE. Primary squamous cell carcinoma of the parotid gland. Arch Otolaryngol Head Neck Surg 1992; 118: 798–801.

84. Gnepp DR, Chen JC, Warren C. Polymorphous low-grade adenocarcinoma of minor salivary gland. An immunohistochemical and clinicopathologic study. Am J Surg Pathol 1988; 12: 461–468.

85. Gnepp DR, Corio RL, Brannon RB. Small cell carcinoma of the major salivary glands. Cancer 1986; 58: 705–714.

86. Gnepp DR, Schroeder W, Heffner D. Synchronous tumors arising in a single major salivary gland. Cancer 1989; 63: 1219–1224.

87. Gnepp DR, Wick MR. Small cell carcinoma of the major salivary glands. An immunohistochemical study. Cancer 1990; 66: 185–192.

88. Goode RK, Corio RL. Oncocytic adenocarcinoma of salivary glands. Oral Surg Oral Med Oral Pathol 1988; 65: 61–66.

89. Granick MS, Erickson ER, Hanna DC. Accuracy of frozen-section diagnosis in salivary gland lesions. Head & Neck Surgery 1985; 7: 465–467.

90. Haan de LD, Mulder de PHM, Vermorken JB, et al. Cisplatin-base chemotherapy in advanced adenoid cystic carcinoma of the head and neck. Head & Neck 1992; 14: 273–277.

91. Hagiwara T, Yoshida H, Takeda Y. Epithelial-myoepithelial carcinoma of a minor salivary gland of the palate. A case report. Int J Oral Maxillofac Surg 1995; 24: 160–161.

92. Hamilton-Dutoit SJ, Hamilton Therkildsen M, Hj gaard Nielsen N, et al. Undifferentiated carcinoma of the salivary gland in Greenlandic Eskimos: Demonstration of Epstein-Barr virus DNA in situ nucleic acid hybridization. Hum Pathol 1991; 22: 811–815.

93. Hamper K, Schimmelpenning H, Caselitz J, et al. Mucoepidermoid tumors of the salivary glands. Correlation of cytophotometrical data and prognosis. Cancer 1989; 63: 708–717.

94. Hamper K. Brügmann M, Koppermann R, et al. Epithelial-myoepithelial duct carcinoma of salivary glands: a follow-up and cytophomometric study of 21 cases. J Oral Pathol Med 1989; 18: 299–304.

95. Hamper K, Mausch H-E, Caselitz J, et al. Acinic cell carcinoma of the salivary glands: The prognostic relevance of DNA cytophotometry in a retrospective study of long duration (1965–1987). Oral Surg Oral Med Oral Pathol 1990; 69: 68–75.

96. Hamper K, Lazar F, Dieter M, et al. Prognostic factors for adenoid cystic carcinoma of the head and neck: a retrospective evaluation of 96 cases. J Oral Pathol Med 1990; 19: 101–107.

97. Hegarty DJ, Hopper C, Speight PM. Inverted ductal papilloma of minor salivary glands. J Oral Pathol Med 1994; 23: 334–336.

98. Hermanek P, Sobin LH. TNM Classification of malignant tumours. 4th ed., 2nd. rev. International Union Against Cancer. Springer-Verlag, Berlin, Heidelberg, New York, 1992.

99. Hicks MJ, El-Naggar AK, Flaitz CM, et al. Histocytologic grading of mucoepidermoid carcinoma of major salivary glands in prognosis and survival: a clinicopathologic and flow cytometric investigation. Head & Neck 1995; 17: 89–95.

100. Hosokawa Y, Ohmori K, Kaneko M, et al. Analysis of adenoid cystic carcinoma treated by radiotherapy. Oral Surg Oral Med Oral Pathol 1992; 74: 251–255.

101. Hsueh C, Gonzalez-Crussi F. Sialoblastoma: A case report and review of the literature on congenital epithelial tumors of salivary gland origin. Pediatric Pathology 1992; 12: 205–214.

102. Hui KK, Luna MA, Batsakis JG, et al. Undifferentiated carcinomas of the major salivary glands. Oral Surg Oral Med Oral Pathol 1990; 69: 76–83.

103. Humphrey PA, Ingram P, Tucker A, et al. Crystalloids in salivary gland pleomorphic adenomas. Arch Pathol Lab Med 1989; 113: 390–393.

104. Huntrakoon M. Neuroendocrine carcinoma of the parotid gland: A report of two cases with ultrastructural and immunohistochemical studies. Hum Pathol 1987; 18: 1212–1217.

105. Hyjek E, Smith WJ, Isaacson PG. Primary B-cell lymphoma of salivary glands and its relationship to myoepithelial sialadenitis. Hum Pathol 1988; 19: 766–776.

106. Ishikawa T, Imada S, Ijuhin N. Intraductal papilloma of the anterior lingual salivary gland. Case report and immunohistochemical study. Int J Oral Maxillofac Surg 1993; 22: 116–117.

107. Jayaram G, Verma AK, Sood N, et al. Fine needle aspiration cytology of salivary gland lesions. J Oral Pathol Med 1994; 23: 256–261.

108. Jie W, Qiguang W, Kaihua S, et al. Quantitative multivariate analysis of myoepithelioma and myoepithelial carcinoma. Int J Oral Maxillofac Surg 1995; 24: 153–157.

109. Jones AS, Phillips DE, Cook JA, et al. A randomised phase II trial of Epirubicin and 5-Fluorouracil versus Cisplatinum in the palliation of advanced and recurrent malignant tumour of the salivary glands. Br J Cancer 1993; 67: 112–114.

110. Kane WJ, McCaffrey TV, Olsen KD, et al. Primary parotid malignancies. A clinical and pathologic review. Arch Otolaryngol Head Neck Surg 1991; 117: 307–315.

111. Kaneda T, Minami M, Ozawa K, et al. Imaging tumors of the minor salivary glands. Oral Surg Oral Med Oral Pathol 1994; 77: 385–390.

112. Kaplan MJ, Johns ME, Cantrall RW. Chemotherapy for salivary gland cancer. Otolaryngol Head Neck Surg 1986; 95: 165–170.

113. Khullar SM, Best PV. Adenomatosis of minor salivary glands. Report of a case. Oral Surg Oral Med Oral Pathol 1992; 74: 783–787.

114. Kim KH, Sung MW, Chung PS, et al. Adenoid cystic carcinoma of the head and neck. Arch Otolaryngol Head Neck Surg 1994; 120: 721–726.

115. Klijanienko J, Micheau C, Bosq J, et al. Analyse histoclinique des cylindromes des glandes salivaires accessoires. A propos de 58 cas suivis a l'Institut Gustave-Roussy. Bull Cancer 1989; 76: 133–143.

116. Koka VN, Tiwari RM, Waal van der I, et al. Adenoid cystic carcinoma of the salivary glands: Clinicopathological survey of 51 patients. J Laryngol Otol 1989; 103: 675–679.

117. Kountakis SE, SooHoo W, Maillard A. Lymphoepithelial carcinoma of the parotid gland. Head & Neck 1995; 17: 445–450.

118. Kurabayashi T, Ida M, Ohbayashi N, et al. Criteria for differentiating superficial from deep lobe tumours of the parotid gland by computed tomography. Dentomaxillofac Radiol 1993; 22: 81–85.

119. Layfield LJ, Tan P, Glasgow BJ. Fine-needle aspiration of salivary gland lesions. Comparison with frozen sections and histologic findings. Arch Pathol Lab Med 1987; 111: 346–353.

120. Lee G, Wong DY-K, Chang RC-S. Hemangiopericytoma of the parotid gland: report of case. J Oral Maxillofac Surg 1992; 50: 1329–1332.

121. Lefor AT, Ord RA. Multiple synchronous bilateral Warthin's tumors of the parotid glands with pleomorphic adenoma. Case report and review of the literature. Oral Surg Oral Med Oral Pathol 1993; 76: 319–324.

122. Lewis JE, Olsen KD, Weiland LH. Acinic cell carcinoma. Clinicopathologic review. Cancer 1991; 67: 172–179.

123. Li X, Tsuji T, Wen S, et al. Cytoplasmic expression of p53 protein and its morphological features in salivary gland lesions. J Oral Pathol Med 1995; 24: 201–205.

124. Licitra L, Marchini S, Spinazzè S, et al. Cisplatin in advanced salivary gland carcinoma. A phase II study of 25 patients. Cancer 1991; 68: 1874–1877.

125. Lo AK, Topf JS, Jackson IT, et al. Minor salivary gland basal cell adenocarcinoma of the palate. J Oral Maxillofac Surg 1992; 50: 531–534.

126. Loy TS, McLaughlin R, Odom LF, et al. Mucoepidermoid carcinoma of the parotid as a second malignant neoplasm in children. Cancer 1989; 64: 2174–2177.

127. Lucarini JW, Sciubba JJ, Khettry U, et al. Terminal duct carcinoma. Recognition of a low-grade salivary adenocarcinoma. Arch Otolaryngol Head Neck Surg 1994; 120: 1010–1015.

128. Luna MA, Tortoledo ME, Allen M. Salivary dermal analogue tumors arising in lymph nodes. Cancer 1987; 59: 1165–1169.

129. Luna MA, El-Naggar EK, Batsakis JG. Flow cytometric DNA content of adenoid cystic carcinoma of submandibular gland. Arch Otolaryngol Head Neck Surg 1990; 116: 1291–1296.

130. Luna MA, Tortoledo ME, Ordóñez NG, et al. Primary sarcomas of the major salivary glands. Arch Otolaryngol Head Neck Surg 1991; 117: 302–306.

131. Mantravadi J, Roth LM, Kafrawy AH. Vascular neoplasms of the parotid gland. Parotid vascular tumors. Oral Surg Oral Med Oral Pathol 1993; 75: 70–75.

132. Martin H, Janda J, Werbs M, et al. Ungewöhnliches, ein pleomorphes Speicheldrüsenadenom imitierendes Chordom der Halsregion. HNO 1990; 38: 462–464.

133. McCluggage G, Sloan J, Cameron S, et al. Basal cell adenocarcinoma of the submandibular gland. Oral Surg Oral Med Oral Pathol 1995; 79: 342–350.

134. McGregor AD, Burgoyne M, Tan KC. Recurrent pleomorphic salivary adenoma – the relevance of age at first presentation. Br J Plast Surg 1988; 41: 177–181.

135. McGuirt WF, Keyes JW, Greven KM, et al. Preoperative identification of benign versus malignant parotid masses: a comparative study including positron emission tomography. Laryngoscope 1995; 105: 579–584.

136. McLoughlin PM, Barrett AW, Speight PM. Oncocytoma of the submandibular gland. Int J Oral Maxillofac Surg 1994; 23: 294–295.

137. McMillan MD, Smith CJ, Smillie AC. Canalicular adenoma: report of five cases with ultrastructural observations. J Oral Pathol Med 1993; 22: 368–373.

138. Medeiros LJ, Rizzi R, Lardelli P, et al. Malignant lymphoma involving a Warthin's tumor: a case with immunophenotypic and gene rearrangement analysis. Hum Pathol 1990; 21: 974–977.

139. Merrick Y, Albeck H, Nielsen NH, et al. Familial clustering of salivary gland carcinoma in Greenland. Cancer 1986; 57: 2097–2102.

140. Miglianico L, Eschwege F, Marandas P, et al. Cervico-facial adenoid cystic carcinoma: study of 102 cases. Influence of radiation therapy. Int J Radiation Oncology Biol Phys 1987; 13: 673–678.

141. Milchgrub S, Gnepp DR, Vuitch F, et al. Hyalinizing clear cell carcinoma of salivary gland. Am J Surg Pathol 1994; 18: 74–82.

142. Miller AS, Hartman GG, Chen S-Y, et al. Estrogen receptor assay in polymorphous low-grade adenocarcinoma and adenoid cystic carcinoma of salivary gland origin. An immunohistochemical study. Oral Surg Oral Med Oral Pathol 1994; 77: 36–40.

143. Miller AS, Harwick RD, Alfaro-Miranda M. Search for correlation of radon levels and incidence of salivary gland tumors. Oral Surg Oral Med Oral Pathol 1993; 75: 58–63.

144. Mini AJ. Acinic cell carcinoma arising in a parotid lymph node. Int J Oral Maxillofac Surg 1993; 22: 289–291.

145. Monk JS, Church JS. Warthin's tumor. A high incidence and no sex predominance in Central Pennsylvania. Arch Otolaryngol Head Neck Surg 1992; 118: 477–478.

146. Morrison GAJ, Shaw HJ. Squamous carcinoma arising within a Warthin's tumour of the parotid gland. J Laryngol Otol 1988; 102: 1189–1191.

147. Mostofi R, Wood RS, Christison W, et al. Low-grade papillary adenocarcinoma of minor salivary glands. Case report and literature review. Oral Surg Oral Med Oral Pathol 1992; 73: 591–595.

148. Murrah VA, Batsakis JG. Salivary duct carcinoma. Ann Otol Rhinol Laryngol 1994; 103: 244–247.

149. Nascimento AG, Amaral ALP, Prado LAF, et al. Mucoepidermoid carcinoma of salivary glands: a clinicopathologic study of 46 cases. Head & Neck Surg 1986; 8: 409–417.

150. Neville BW, Damm DD, Weir JC, et al. Labial salivary gland tumors. Cancer 1988; 61: 2113–2116.

151. Ng WK, Ma L. Pleomorphic adenoma with extensive lipometaplasia. Histopathology 1995; 27: 285–288.

152. Nitsche N, Waitz G, Iro H. Darstellung von Erkrankungen der Glandula parotis durch hochauflösende Magnetresonanztomographie. HON 1990; 38: 451–456.

153. Ogawa I, Miyauchi M, Takata T, et al. Proliferative activity of salivary gland pleomorphic adenomas and myoepitheliomas as evaluated by the proliferating cell nuclear antigen (PCNA) labeling index (LI). J Oral Pathol Med 1993; 22: 447–450.

154. Önder T, Tiwari RM, Waal van der I, et al. Malignant adenolymphoma of the parotid gland: report of carcinomatous transformation. J Laryngol Otol 1990; 104: 656–661.

155. Osaki T, Hirota J, Ohno A, et al. Mucinous adenocarcinoma of the submandibular gland. Cancer 1990; 66: 1796–1801.

156. Owens RM, Friedman CD, Becker SP. Renal cell carcinoma with metastasis to the parotid gland: case reports and review of the literature. Head & Neck 1989; 11: 174–178.

157. Palmer TJ, Gleeson MJ, Eveson JW, et al. Oncocytic adenomas and oncocytic hyperplasia of salivary glands: a clinicopathologic study of 26 cases. Histopathology 1990; 16: 476–493.

158. Pedersen D, Overgaard J, S gaard H, et al. Malignant parotid tumors in 110 consecutive patients: treatment results and prognosis. Laryngoscope 1992; 102: 1064–1069.

159. Phillips PP, Olsen KD. Recurrent pleomorphic adenoma of the parotid gland: report of 126 cases and a review of the literature. Ann Otol Rhinol Laryngol 1995; 104: 100–104.

160. Preston-Martin S, Thomas DC, White SC, et al. Prior exposure to medical and dental X-rays related to tumors of the parotid gland. J Nat Cancer Inst 1988; 80: 943–949.

161. Raustia AM, Oikarinen KS, Luotonen J, et al. Parotid gland carcinoma simulating signs and symptoms of craniomandibular disorders – a case report. J Craniomandibular practice 1993; 11: 153–156.

162. Rigual NR, Milley P, Loré JM, et al. Accuracy of frozen-section diagnosis in salivary gland neoplasms. Head & Neck Surgery 1986; 8: 442–446.

163. Ritland F, Lubensky I, LiVolsi VA. Polymorphous low-grade adenocarcinoma of the parotid salivary gland. Arch Pathol Lab Med 1993; 117: 1261–1263.

164. Sakashita H, Miyata M, Miyamoto H, et al. Glomus tumor originating in the parotid rgeion. J Oral Maxillofac Surg 1995; 53: 830–834.

165. Scher RL, Feldman PS, Levine PA. Small-cell carcinoma of the parotid gland with neuroendocrine features. Arch Otolaryngol Head Neck Surg 1988; 114: 319–321.

166. Schilling JA, Block BL, Speigel JC. Synchronous unilateral parotid neoplasms of different histologic types. Head & Neck 1989; 11: 179–183.

167. Seifert G. Klassifikation der mesenchymalen Tumoren der grossen Speicheldrüsen. Dtsch Z Mund Kiefer GesichtsChir 1988; 12: 64–73.

168. Seifert G. WHO International Histological Classification of Tumours. Histological Typing of Salivary Gland Tumours. 2nd ed. Springer-Verlag; Berlin, Heidelberg, New York, 1991.

169. Seifert G. Histopathology of malignant salivary gland tumours. Oral Oncol, Eur J Cancer 1992; 28B: 49–56.

170. Seifert G, Sobin LH. The World Health Organizations's Histological Classification of Salivary Gland Tumors. Cancer 1992; 70: 379–385.

171. Shemen LJ, Huvos AG, Spiro RH. Squamous cell carcinoma of salivary gland origin. Head & Neck Surg 1987; 9: 235–240.

172. Shick PC, Riordan GP, Foss RD. Estrogen and progesterone receptors in salivary gland adenoid cystic carcinoma. Oral Surg Oral Med Oral Pathol 1995; 80: 440–444.

173. Shingaki S, Ohtake K, Nomura T, et al. The role of radiotherapy in the management of salivary gland carcinomas. J Cranio-Max-Fac Surg 1992; 20: 220–224.

174. Simpson RHW, Clarke TJ, Sarsfield PTL, et al. Salivary duct adenocarcinoma. Histopathology 1991; 18: 229–235.

175. Simpson RHW, Clarke TJ, Sarsfield PTL, et al. Polymorphous low-grade adenocarcinoma of the salivary glands: a clinicopathological comparison with adenoid cystic carcinoma. Histopathology 1991; 19: 121–129.

176. Simpson RHW, Sarsfield PTL, Clarke T, et al. Clear cell carcinoma of minor salivary glands. Histopathology 1990; 17: 433–438.

177. Slootweg PJ. Low-grade adenocarcinoma of the oral cavity: polymorphous or papillary. J Oral Pathol Med 1993; 23: 327–330.

178. Soini Y, Kamel D, Nuorva K, et al. Low p53 protein expression in salivary gland tumours compared with lung carcinomas. Virchows Archiv A Pathol Anat 1992; 421: 415–420.

179. Spiro IJ, Wang CC, Montgomery WW. Carcinoma of the parotid gland. Analysis of treatment results and patterns of failure after combined surgery and radiation therapy. Cancer 1993; 71: 2699–2705.

180. Spiro RH. Salivary neoplasms: overview of a 35-year experience with 2,807 patients. Head & Neck Surg 1986; 8: 177–184.

181. Spiro RH, Armstrong J, Harrison L, et al. Carcinoma of major salivary glands. Recent trends. Arch Otolaryngol Head Neck Surg 1989; 115: 316–321.

182. Spitz MR, Tilley BC, Batsakis JG, et al. Risk factors for major salivary gland carcinoma. A case-comparison study. Cancer 1984; 54: 1854–1859.

183. Spitz MR, Fueger JJ, Goepfert H, et al. Salivary gland cancer. A case-control investigation of risk factors. Arch Otolaryngol Head Neck Surg 1990; 116: 1163–1166.

184. Suei Y, Tanimoto K, Taguchi A, et al. Radiographic evaluation of bone invasion of adenoid cystic carcinoma in the oral and maxillofacial region. J Oral Maxillofac Surg 1994; 52: 821–826.

185. Szanto PA, Luna MA, Tortoledo E, et al. Histologic grading of adenoid cystic carcinoma of the salivary glands. Cancer 1984; 54: 1062–1069.

186. Takahashi H, Tsuda N, Tezuka F, et al. Non-Hodgkin's lymphoma of the major salivary gland: a morphologic and immunohistochemical study of 15 cases. J Oral Pathol Med 1990; 19: 306–312.

187. Takata T, Ogawa I, Nikai H. Sebaceous carcinoma of the parotid gland. An immunohistochemical and ultrastructral study. Virchows Archiv A Pathol Anat 1989; 414: 459–464.

188. Takeda Y. Crystalloid granuloma of the parotid gland: a previously undescribed salivary gland lesion. J Oral Pathol Med 1991; 20: 234–236.

189. Tateishi A, Nodai T, Fukuyama H, et al. Primary mucoepidermoid carcinoma of an intraparotid lymph node. J Oral Maxillfoac Surg 1992; 50: 535–538.

190. Thomas KM, Hutt MSR, Borgstein J. Salivary gland tumors in Malawi. Cancer 1980; 46: 2328–2334.

191. Timon CI, Dardick I, Panzarella T, et al. Acinic cell carcinoma of salivary glands. Prognostic relevance of DNA flow cytometry and nucleolar organizer regions. Arch Otolaryngol Head Neck Surg 1994; 120: 727–730.

192. Tischendorf L, Herrmann PK, Luttermann Th. Konsequenzen aus Studien zur Reklassifizierung von Geschwülsten der Kopfspeicheldrüsen. Dtsch Z Mund Kiefer GesichtsChir 1991; 15: 35–37.

193. Traxler M. Hajek P, Solar P, et al. Magnetic resonance in lesions of the parotid gland. Int J Oral Maxillofac Surg 1991; 20: 170–174.

194. Vincent SD, Hammond HL, Finkelstein MW. Clinical and therapeutic features of polymorphous low-grade adenocarcinoma. Oral Surg Oral Med Oral Pathol 1994; 77: 41–47.

195. Vrielinck LJG, Ostyn F, Van Damme B, et al. The significance of perineural spread in adenoid cystic carcinoma of the major and minor salivary glands. Int J Oral Maxillofac Surg 1988; 17: 190–193.

196. Vuhahula EAM, Nikai H, Ogawa I, et al. Correlation between argyrophilic nucleolar organizer region (AgNOR) counts and histologic grades with respect to biologic behavior of salivary adenoid cystic carcinoma. J Oral Pathol Med 1995; 24: 437–442.

197. Wal van der JE, Snow GB, Waal van der I. Histological reclassification of 101 intraoral salivary gland tumours (new WHO classifcation). J Clin Pathol 1992; 45: 834–835.

198. Wal van der JE, Snow GB, Karim ABMF, et al. Adenoid cystic carcinoma of the palate with squamous metaplasia or basaloid-squamous carcinoma? Report of a case. J Oral Pathol Med 1994; 23: 461–464.

199. Wal van der JE, Carter RL, Klijanienko J, et al. Histologic re-evaluation of 101 intraoral salivary gland tumors by an EORTC-study group. J Oral Pathol Med 1993; 22: 21–22.

200. Wal van der JE, Davids JJ, Waal van der I. Extraparotid Warthin's tumours – report of 10 cases. Br J Oral Maxillofac Surg 1993; 31: 43–44.

201. Wal van der JE, Snow GB, Karim ABMF, et al. Intraoral adenoid cystic carcinoma: the role of postoperative radiotherapy in local control. Head & Neck 1989; 11: 497–499.

202. Wal van der JE, Waal van der I. The rare sialadenoma papilliferum. Report of a case and review of the literature. Int J Oral Maxillofac Surg 1992; 21: 104–106.
203. Waldron CA, El-Mofty SK, Gnepp DR. Tumors of the intraoral minor salivary glands: A demographic and histologic study of 426 cases. Oral Surg Oral Med Oral Pathol 1988; 66: 323–333.
204. Warfield AT, Smallman LA. Simultaneous bilateral pleomorphic adenomas of the parotid glands with unilateral tyrosine rich crystalloids. J Clin Pathol 1994; 47: 362–364.
205. Weber RS, Byers RM, Petit B, et al. Submandibular gland tumors. Adverse histologic factors and therapeutic implications. Arch Otolaryngol Head Neck Surg 1990; 116: 1055–1060.
206. Wenig BM. Hitchcock CL, Ellis GL, et al. Metastasizing mixed tumor of salivary glands. A clinicopathologic and flow cytometric analysis. Am J Surg Pathol 1992; 16: 845–858.
207. Williams SB, Foss RD, Ellis GL. Inflammatory pseudotumors of the major salivary glands. Clinicopathologic and immunohistochemical analysis of six cases. Am J Surg Pathol 1992; 16: 896–902.
208. Williams MD, Pearson MH, Thomas FD. Pilomatrixoma: a rare condition in the differential diagnosis of a parotid swelling. Br J Oral Maxillofac Surg 1991: 23; 201–203.
209. Witten J, Hybert F, Hansen HS. Treatment of malignant tumors in the parotid glands. Cancer 1990; 65: 2515–2520.
210. Woodwards RT, Shepherd NA, Hensher R. Malignant melanoma of the parotid gland: a case report and literature review Br J Oral Maxillofac Surg 1993; 31: 313–315.
211. Xie X, Stenersen TC, Larsen PL, et al. Prognostic value of nuclear volume in adenoid cystic carcinoma of the head and neck. Oncology Reports 1994; 1: 427–432.
212. Yang L, Liu B, Qin C, et al. Comparison of proliferating cell nuclear antigen index in benign and malignant salivary pleomorphic adenoma. Oral Oncol, Eur J Cancer 1994; 30B: 56–60.
213. Young JA. Diagnostic problems in fine needle aspiration cytopathology of the salivary glands. J Clin Pathol 1994; 47: 193–198.
214. Zachariades N, Koumoura F, Liapi-Avgeri G, et al. Extraskeletal Ewing's sarcoma of the parotid regimen: a case report with the detection of the tumour immunophenotypical characteristics. Br J Oral Maxillofac Surg 1994; 32: 328–331.
215. Zurrida S, Alasio L, Tradati N, et al. Fine-needle aspiration of parotid masses. Cancer 1993; 72: 2306–2311.

6 Miscellaneous Lesions and Conditions

6.1 Diagnostic Value of Saliva

There is a good correlation between plasma and saliva levels of a number of hormones and medications. This correlation forms the basis for proposals to use saliva collection as a noninvasive means of monitoring hormones and both therapeutic and illicit drugs. Saliva collection is also being tested at present as a means of screening for the presence of antibodies to human immunodeficiency virus (HIV)-1.

In a review article, the various clinical situations in which salivary analysis can provide valuable information, have been discussed [61]. These include the following:

- Digitalis toxicity
- Affective disorders
- Stomatitis in cancer chemotherapy
- Immunodeficiency of secretory immunoglobulin A (IgA)
- Cigarette smoking
- Dietary nitrates, nitrites, and gastric cancer
- Ovulation time

For instance, concentration of salivary prostaglandins is significantly higher in patients with major depressive disorders than in healthy controls [79].

Salivary cotinine is a reliable indicator of exposure to tobacco smoking [25]; it correlates with urinary levels and with the number of cigarettes smoked per day [56]. Another possible application is the measurement of mercury that is released from amalgam fillings in teeth [80].

Saliva may also be used for monitoring lipid-soluble unconjugated steroids, such as cortisol, aldosterone, and testosterone.

Salivary insulin measurement may also be of clinical relevance [63]. Adrenal stress response to dental treatment could, for example, be measured by a salivary cortisol assay [70].

Therapeutic drug monitoring in saliva is another recent development. It is especially useful when the saliva to plasma concentration ratio is constant over a wide range [61].

In addition to measuring antibodies, e.g., in HIV-positive patients, it is possible to identify a number of specific viral antigens in saliva [33, 61, 102].

6.2 Benign Lymphoepithelial Lesion

6.2.1 Definition

Benign lymphoepithelial lesion (BLEL), also called myoepithelial sialoadenitis (MESA), is a histopathologic entity that is characterized by atrophy of salivary gland parenchyma and lymphocytic infiltration with islands of epithelial and myoepithelial cells replacing the intralobular ducts. The term Mikulicz's disease was previously used to describe the condition.

The adjective "benign" has often been placed in parentheses since the benign character of the lesion is not always clear. It has been stated that, in the presence of a monoclonal B cell population, a diagnosis of BLEL is inappropriate [29]. Others have argued that monoclonality is not necessarily indicative of lymphoma [32]. Furthermore, a few cases of malignant lymphoepithelioma in the parotid gland have been reported [6, 15]; the term "carcinoma ex lymphoepithelial lesion" seems more appropriate [10].

BLEL is more or less limited to the parotid gland and is often found in association with Sjögren's syndrome (see Chap. 3). A rare case of BLEL of the hard palate has been reported [64]; a single case of involvement of the sublingual gland has also been reported [4].

6.2.2 Etiology

The etiology and pathogenesis of BLEL are not well understood. The lesion may be part of Sjögren's syndrome and can be associated with HIV infection.

6.2.3 Epidemiology

BLEL are seen more often in women than in men and usually after the fifth or sixth decade.

6.2.4 Clinical Aspects

The clinical presentation of BLEL is an often asymptomatic, rather diffuse swelling of the parotid gland, sometimes occurring bilaterally (Fig. 6.1). The swelling can be of a recurrent nature.

In some patients, there is a history of recent illness or discomfort. Xerostomia may or may not be present.

The use of sialography and scintigraphy in obtaining a correct diagnosis is of limited value. Aspiration cytology may be a useful diagnostic tool and may even differentiate between BLEL and malignant lymphoreticular disease. The final diagnosis can be made only by histopathologic examination, which often requires a superficial parotidectomy.

6.2.5 Histological Aspects

The disease is characterized histologically by the replacement of parenchymal salivary gland structures with a dense lymphocytic infil-

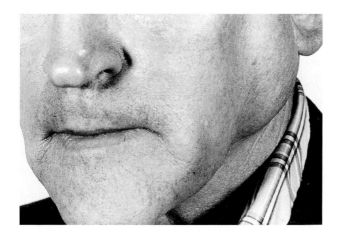

Fig. 6.1. Diffuse swelling of parotid gland caused by a benign lymphoepithelial lesion

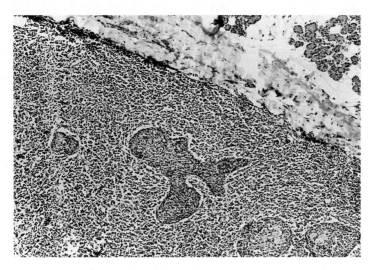

Fig. 6.2. Low-power view of benign lymphoepithelial lesion. Note the epimyo-epithelial islands in the lymphoid tissue

trate in which epimyo-epithelial islands are encountered. These islands most likely represent persisting ducts of which the epithelial lining may show extensive proliferation even to the extent of obliterating the lumen (Fig. 6.2). In long-standing lesions, hyaline material can be encountered in the epithelial islands. This material apparently consists of basement membrane material [81].

The presence of epimyo-epithelial islands is important in making a final diagnosis of BLEL. In the absence of such islands, a diagnosis of malignant lymphoreticular disease is more likely [44]. Carcinomatous changes in the epimyo-epithelial islands are rare. Some refer to this entity as malignant lymphoepithelial lesion (MLEL). A high incidence of MLEL among Eskimos has been reported [52].

Patients with BLEL who also suffer from the sicca syndrome, leukopenia, or hypogammaglobulinemia may have an increased risk of developing malignant lymphoreticular disease.

6.2.6 Treatment

Treatment, if indicated for cosmetic reasons or because of diagnostic purposes, consists of a superficial or even a total parotidectomy with facial nerve preservation [37]. Recurrence is rare.

6.3 Developmental Disturbances

6.3.1 Agenesis, Aplasia, and Hypoplasia

Agenesis, aplasia, and hypoplasia of the major salivary glands and/or their excretory ducts (absence of an extretory duct is termed "atresia") are extremely rare [23, 27, 50, 53]. The disturbance may occur in isolation or in conjunction with other developmental anomalies, such as absence of the lacrimal glands. Some authors have reported familial salivary gland aplasia [108].

Since symptoms are not always present, the condition may go unnoticed. On the other hand, rampant caries and marked xerostomia may lead to the detection of aplasia of one or more major salivary glands [77].

6.3.2 Hyperplasia

Occasionally, hyperplastic salivary gland tissue may be encountered, particularly on the palate, with the clinical appearance of a neoplasm (Fig. 6.3) [9]. In case of multifocal hyperplasia of the intraoral salivary glands, the term adenomatosis oris is sometimes used. The latter term has also been used to describe the multifocal occurrence of benign tumors of salivary glands, particularly in the lips [51].

The etiology of hyperplasia is unknown. There is no distinct sex or age preference [83]. Wide surgical excision is the treatment of choice.

6.3.3 Ectopic Salivary Glands

Ectopic salivary glands (salivary "choristomas") may occur in the neck. In such cases, the clinical presentation is usually that of a cystic mass or a draining sinus in the anterolateral neck. Diagnosis requires both histological verification of salivary tissue and a location remote from the major and minor salivary glands [75].

Ectopic salivary glands may also occur within the jaws, particularly in the mandible. In the latter location, the salivary gland tissue is thought to be enclosed during embryological development (see also Sect. 6.3.4). Another possible explanation is a differentiation from

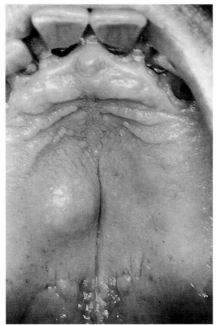

a

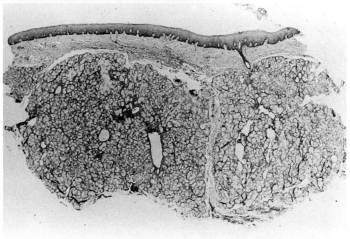

b

Fig. 6.3. a Firm, elastic swelling near the palatal midline. **b** The biopsy showed the presence of normal salivary tissue, compatible with the diagnosis of salivary gland hyperplasia

primitive epithelial rests of either odontogenic or nonodontogenic origin. Ectopic salivary glands have also been reported to occur on the buccal aspect of the upper alveolar ridge and the anterior mandibular gingivae and in a variety of other locations such as the middle ear, the hypophysis, and the thyroid gland.

6.3.4 Lingual Mandibular Salivary Gland Depression Cyst

Lingual mandibular salivary gland depression cyst, Stafne cyst, latent or static bone cyst, and lingual cortical defect of the mandible are all used synonymously. The "cyst" represents a concavity of the lingual aspect of the mandibular bone or, rarely, a cavity within the bone due to the enclosure of salivary gland tissue during the embryonic stage. However, the phenomenon has also been ascribed to a resorptive process caused by hyperplasia of salivary gland tissue, to an anomaly in the facial artery, or to functional adaptation of the bone.

The prevalence is estimated to be about 0.1%–0.4%. The defect is much more common in men than in women, and occurrence in children is rare.

The cyst is asymptomatic and is almost invariably detected as an incidental finding on the radiograph, especially since the availability of panoramic radiographs.

Radiographically, the defect is round to oval and is almost always located near the angle of the mandible, usually inferior to the mandibular canal (Fig. 6.4). Location above the mandibular canal is rare. Some lesions have been reported in the anterior region of the mandible. Anterior lingual mandibular salivary gland defects are rare [8]. Bilateral occurrence is exceptional, as is a bilocular or multilocular appearance. In rare instances, the location of the defect may mimic the presence of an odontogenic cyst, e.g., a dentigerous cyst of a wisdom tooth.

The cyst may vary in size from a few millimeters up to several centimeters. The radiolucency is partially or completely surrounded by a dense radiopaque line.

Chen and Ohba [17] have proposed a classification system of these defects based on the position and location of lesions relative to the mandibular canal and the cortical plate of the border of the mandible.

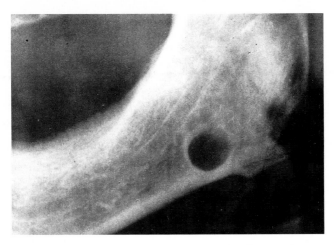

Fig. 6.4. Characteristic radiographic appearance of lingual mandibular salivary gland depression cyst

In the majority of the surgically explored cases, salivary gland tissue was encountered. The presence of lymphoid tissue or a lymph node has also been reported.

The absence of symptoms, site specificity, and the radiographic appearance are usually sufficient for the final diagnosis, making surgical exploration redundant. Surgical exploration is indicated only when the nature of the lesion remains unclear on clinical and radiographic grounds. No follow-up is required.

6.4 Frey's Syndrome

In approximately 10%–20% of parotidectomies, Frey's syndrome (also called auriculotemporal syndrome or gustatory sweating) develops, consisting of redness and sweating of the skin in the surgical field during meals. These signs can be quite annoying for the patient.

Gustatory sweating as the result of the surgical removal of a submandibular gland is rare [39]. Occasionally, bilateral gustatory sweating is observed in patients with no history of facial trauma or surgery [68].

Parasympatic fibers are apparently misdirected during their regeneration, resulting in a sympathetically driven vasomotor effect of sweating and flushing of the skin. The Minor starch-iodine test can be used to delineate the precise area of sweating (Fig. 6.5) [89].

Daily topical application of 1%–2% glycopyrrolate (an anticholinergic agent) may be quite helpful [42, 66]. Another anticholinergic agent, 2% diphemanil methylsulfate, applied topically every other day may be useful [54]. Others have used aluminum trichloride hexahydrate gel [14, 89]. In rare instances, surgical intervention may be required [7]. Recently, the effectiveness of intracutaneously injected botulinum toxin A has been demonstrated in 14 patients [26]. The toxin ($0.5\,U/cm^2$) was injected into the affected skin area as determined by the Minor starch-iodine test mentioned above. Gustatory sweating in the treated skin area ceased completely within 2 days and did not reappear during a maximum follow-up of 13 months.

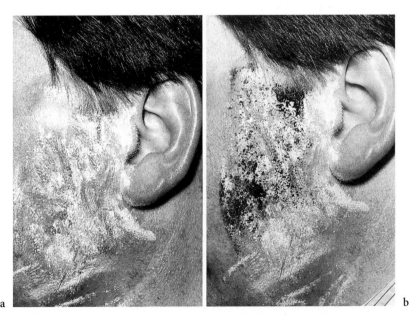

a   b

Fig. 6.5. a Starch-iodine test in patient suffering from Frey's syndrome. **b** Six minutes after gustatory stimulation

6.5 Necrotizing Sialometaplasia

6.5.1 Definition

The term necrotizing sialometaplasia (NS) was introduced in 1973 by Abrams et al. [1] to describe a reactive necrotizing disease of the salivary glands, which mainly occurs in the minor salivary glands. A few hundred cases have been reported since this description [16]. Furthermore, NS can be observed in tissues of the nasal cavity and paranasal sinuses, as well as in the major salivary glands [11].

Squamous/mucinous metaplasia of oncocytic tumors appears to be related only morphologically to necrotizing sialometaplasia [100]. One case of proliferative sialometaplasia arising in an intraparotid lymph node has been reported [35], but no other such cases have been published.

6.5.2 Etiology

NS is believed to have a vascular-based infarct genesis. In many cases of NS, the history reveals a recent trauma, biopsy, or local injection of an anesthetic solution containing a vasoconstrictor [106]. Infarction due to the vasoconstrictive action of the injection fluid seems to be the most likely cause in such cases.

6.5.3 Epidemiology

In a review of the literature, a slight male predominance is found [16]. The average age at diagnosis is approximately 45 years.

6.5.4 Clinical Aspects

NS may occur everywhere in the oral cavity. However, the junction of the hard and soft palate is the site of predilection. The clinical presentation in the case of palatal involvement is either an ulcer or

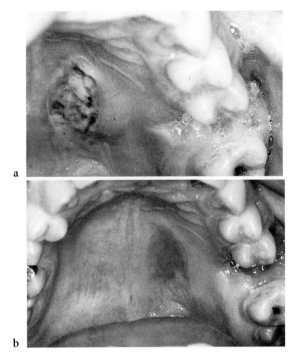

a

b

Fig. 6.6. a Palatal ulceration 1 week after injection of a local anaesthetic solution. A biopsy showed the histological features of necrotizing sialometaplasia. **b** No treatment was instituted, and spontaneous healing took place in 3 weeks

a swelling, sometimes bilateral, with an initially intact mucosa (Fig. 6.6). The size may vary from a few millimeters up to more than 1 cm. The underlying bone remains intact. The lesions are usually painful.

There are no clinical features that are diagnostic of NS. When dealing with an ulcer or a swelling of the palate, one should therefore include a number of lesions in the differential diagnosis, such as salivary gland tumor, malignant lymphoreticular disease, and also, in the absence of any pigmentation, an amelanotic melanoma. The possibility of a midline granuloma should also be taken into account, although in this conditon perforation of the palatal bone usually occurs at an early stage. A rare case of NS in a patient with sickle cell anemia has been published [58].

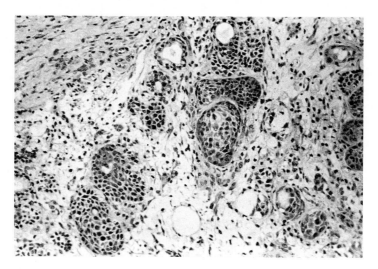

Fig. 6.7. Low-power view of necrotizing sialometaplasia. Necrosis of parenchymal salivary cells and persisting excretory ducts, showing squamous metaplasia

6.5.5 Histological Aspects

The histological picture of NS is characterized by necrosis of the parenchymal cells. The lobular architecture of the involved gland usually remains intact. There may be a mild, lymphoplasma cellular infiltrate. The numerous excretory ducts persist and may show considerable squamous metaplasia of their lining epithelium, occasionally completely obliterating the lumen. A few mitotic figures may be encountered (Fig. 6.7).

Several cases of misinterpretation of NS as squamous cell carcinoma, adenocarcinoma, and mucoepidermoid carcinoma have been reported [69]. On the other hand, NS may obscure an underlying malignant mesenchymal neoplasm [85].

6.5.6 Treatment

The lesion does not require treatment and heals spontaneously in a few weeks.

6.6 Parotid and Submandibular Fistula

Salivary fistulas almost exclusively occur in relation to the parotid gland or its excretory duct (Fig. 6.8). A submandibular salivary gland fistula is rare [95].

Traumatic injury of the face is the most common cause. Occasionally, a salivary fistula may be created during the removal of a skin lesion overlying Stensen's duct. The obstruction of the parotid duct by a calculus may also result in formation of a facial sinus [22]. A rare case of bilateral parotid duct fistula in a 12-year-old boy has been reported in the literature [49]. Furthermore, a case of a parotid fistula has been reported that drained into the maxillary sinus, thereby producing rhinorrhea [30].

Most parotid fistulas heal spontaneously in a few weeks. In persistent cases, an attempt can be made to intraorally dissect the proximal part of the excretory duct and to create a new outlet into the oral cavity. There is rarely a need for the use of salivary flow-decreasing drugs such as atropine or artifical damage of the salivary gland by irradiation.

6.7 Pneumoparotis

Pneumoparotis, also referred to as pneumoparotid, pneumoparotitis, pneumatocele, or wind parotitis, may occur within a few hours fol-

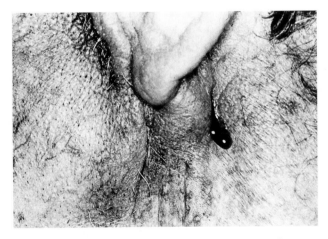

Fig. 6.8. Parotid fistula. (Courtesy of Dr. H.A. Kraaijenhagen, Netherlands)

lowing a surgical procedure using general anaesthesia ("surgical mumps" or "anesthesia mumps") [36]. Bilateral occurrence is rare.

The exact mechanism is unknown. A combination of neuromuscular blocking agents, belladonna drugs, and straining or coughing at the time of extubation seems a reasonable explanation in most cases. However, pneumoparotis can also be caused by dental air instruments through retrograde insufflation of air up Stensen's duct [84, 99]. The onset of the emphysema usually occurs either during the dental treatment or within 1h postoperatively. Other etiologies include glass-blowing, balloon-blowing, and the playing of wind instruments, such as the trumpet or horn. An unusual case of pneumoparotis has been reported that involved background swelling of the parotids because of the respiratory effort required in chronic obstructive pulmonary disease and acute exacerbations associated with episodes of coughing [21]. A few cases of self-induced pneumoparotis in children have been reported [34].

In the case published by Piette and Walker [84], the accumulation of air in the parotid region was shown by X-ray examination. In the case reported by Takenoshita et al. [99], the air in the parotid gland was shown on an echogram.

It is advisable to administer antibiotics for about 1 week. The salivary gland enlargement usually disappears spontaneously within a few days.

6.8 Salivary Gland Involvement in Systemic Diseases

6.8.1 Salivary Gland Involvement in Human Immunodeficiency Virus Infection

Bilateral or unilateral enlargement of the parotid gland has been noted in patients who are seropositive for antibodies to HIV [55, 92]. The term HIV-associated salivary gland disease (HIV-SGD) is often used. It is a relatively common phenomenon in HIV-infected children and is often associated with decreased salivary flow.

The swelling may be painful. A characteristic cystic appearance has been noted in these lesions on clinical and radiographic examination (Figs. 6.9, 6.10) [59]. While clinical symptoms are similar to Sjögren's syndrome, patients with HIV-SGD lack circulating anti-SS-A/Ro and

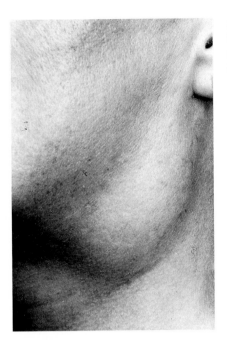

Fig. 6.9. Parotid swelling in human immunodeficiency virus (HIV)-infected patient. (Courtesy of Prof. Dr. G.B. Snow, Netherlands)

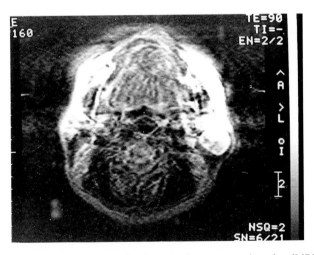

Fig. 6.10. Axial T2-weighted magnetic resonance imaging (MRI) of the same patient as in Fig. 6.9, showing lesion in left parotid gland; note the high and inhomogeneous signal intensity. (Courtesy of Dr. J.A. Castelijns, Netherlands)

anti-SS-B/La [5]. Histologically, a benign lymphoepithelial infiltrate with cystic degeneration is found in parotid specimens from these patients [19, 31, 88, 94, 97, 101]. Presence of a malignant non-Hodgkin's lymphoma has also been reported [20, 45].

Low-dose radiation (8–10 Gy) provides reliable, but only temporary cosmetic palliation in HIV-SGD patients; higher initial doses of radiation may be required to prolong palliation and eliminate recurrences [12].

6.8.2 Cytomegalic Inclusion Disease

In the majority of patients with a positive serological reaction to cytomegalovirus (CMV, one of the herpesviruses), clinical symptoms are absent. The infection seems to occur mainly before birth via the placenta or shortly after birth. CMV can affect the normal maturation of the fetusm and premature birth is not uncommon. The virus shows a predilection for the salivary glands, but may affect other organs as well [96].

The main symptoms of generalized cytomegalic inclusion disease in a newborn are sialadenitis (often parotitis), hepatosplenomegaly, jaundice, anemia, and neurological disturbances. In the majority of adults, antibodies against the virus can be demonstrated in the serum. Reactivation of CMV almost exclusively occurs in immunosuppressed patients.

The diagnosis of the cytomegalic inclusion disease is based on the demonstration of CMV antibodies in the urinary sediment or the saliva, on the histological features (i.e., intranuclear inclusion bodies and epithelial giant cells; Fig. 6.11), on a positive complement-binding reaction, or by the demonstration of an increase in the specific IgM antibody in the serum to at least 1:64. Fine-needle aspiration cytology of a parotid swelling may also lead to a diagnosis of CMV [86]. There is no effective treatment available.

6.8.3 Salivary Gland Involvement in Other Systemic Diseases

A labial or a palatal biopsy may be helpful in establishing the diagnosis of a systemic disease such as *amyloidosis* [18], *sarcoidosis* [62, 76,

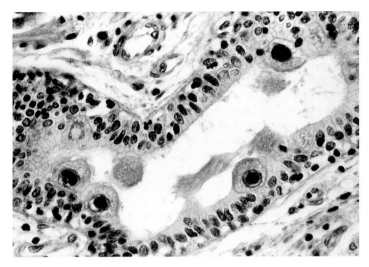

Fig. 6.11. Intranuclear inclusion bodies in the epithelial lining of salivary duct, characteristic of cytomegalic inclusion disease

105], *Wegener's granulomatosis* [72], *Crohn's disease* [90], or *Sjögren's syndrome* (see Chap. 3). A biopsy of the sublingual salivary gland has also been used for this purpose [2]. The sialographic features in these diseases are usually not typical.

In patients with *rheumatoid arthritis* or *systemic lupus erythematosus*, a significant increase in the density of IgG cells within the salivary glands is found [65]. The altered salivary composition in systemic lupus erythematosus might indicate a subclinical involvement of salivary glands in these patients [13].

A rare case of submandibular salivary gland involvement in *hemochromatosis* has been published [24].

Apart from increased salivary gland adiposity in alcoholic cirrhosis, there is no general salivary structural abnormality associated with chronic alcohol abuse [91].

Heerfordt's syndrome, also called uveoparotitis, is an extremely rare syndrome characterized by anterior uveitis, parotitis, and paralysis of the facial nerve. The syndrome is currently considered to be a subacute type of sarcoidosis.

In rare instances, enlargement of the major salivary glands may be caused by *Wegener's granulomatosis* [72]. Furthermore, a case of a localized primary *amyloid* tumor of the parotid gland has been reported [98].

6.9 Sialadenosis

6.9.1 Definition

The term sialadenosis refers to a non inflammatory parenchymatous disease of the major salivary glands caused by a secretory and metabolic disturbance of the acinar parenchyma.

6.9.2 Etiology

Sialadenosis may actually be considered to be the result of a peripheral autonomic neuropathy and can be associated with hormonal disturbances, such as thyroid insufficiency, malnutrition, alcohol abuse, disorders of the nervous system, liver cirrhosis, and mucoviscidosis. Nutritional chronic sialadenosis, probably due to excessive potato consumption, has been reported from the Highlands of Papua New Guinea [71]. Bilateral parotid swelling may also occur in infants recovering from kwashiorkor. The condition has also been reported to be the result of the use of certain drugs. Bulimia and anorexia nervosa have been implicated as possible causes of transient salivary gland hypertrophy [38, 40, 60, 78].

6.9.3 Clinical Aspects

In most cases the parotid glands are involved, often bilaterally (Fig. 6.12), and in rare instances the submandibular glands are also involved. The swellings are painless and may be of a recurrent nature. The patient may complain of fatigue.

In most instances, the diagnosis sialadenosis is based on the medical history and the clinical signs and symptoms. The sialogram shows a very thin structure of the ducts (Fig. 6.13).

In the early stage, computed tomography (CT) scans show only enlargement of the glands. In the later stages, the density of the glandular tissue is reduced.

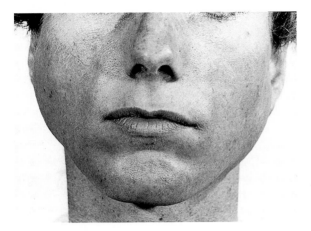

Fig. 6.12. Bilateral parotid swelling caused by sialadenosis

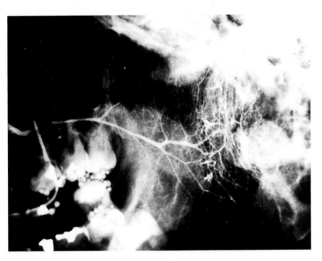

Fig. 6.13. Sialogram of parotid gland in patient with sialadenosis. Note the thin, delicate pattern of ducts

6.9.4 Cytological and Histological Aspects

The need for cytological or histopathologic examination is question-able because of the often inconspicious appearance, consisting of hypertrophy of the acinar cells with or without degranulation and, in a later stage, lipomatosis. However, the presence of lipomatosis with the partial replacement of functional parenchymal cells by fat and connective tissue seems merely to represent an age-related change [107]. Nevertheless, cytological examination may be helpful for ruling out other lesions or conditions.

Histologically, the diameter of acinar cells in sialadenosis may be up to two to three times the normal diameter. The nuclei are displaced toward the basal part of the cell, and inflammatory cells are absent [93]. In spite of the apparently clear description of the histological aspects in the literature, the diagnosis of sialadenosis is difficult to arrive at by histological examination alone.

6.9.5 Treatment

Treatment is primarily directed toward the detection of a possible underlying disorder, e.g., functional disturbances of the pancreas, liver, kidneys, and thyroid. Only in the case of cosmetic disfigurement, and in the absence of an underlying disorder, may a parotidectomy be considered.

6.10 Sialolithiasis

6.10.1 Definition

Calculus formation in the salivary glands or its excretory ducts is known as sialolithiasis. It usually occurs in the form of a solitary concrement, varying in size from less than 1 mm up to several centimeters.

Sialoliths consist of mineral substances and organic material.

6.10.2 Etiology

The exact etiology and pathogenesis are unknown. Theories include calcification around foreign bodies, desquamated epithelial cells, and inflammatory changes in the duct. There is no distinct relationship with other systemic disorders. However, there may be a relationship with nephrolithiasis [57].

6.10.3 Epidemiology

There is a slight predilection for occurrence in men [57], and patients are usually above the age of 40 years.

6.10.4 Clinical Aspects

The majority of sialoliths are located in the excretory duct of the submandibular glands, probably due to the mucin content and the high Ca^{2+} content when compared with the parotid gland (Fig. 6.14). The calculus formation sometimes takes place in the submandibular gland itself. Occurrence in the parotid gland is quite rare, as is calculus formation in the intraoral salivary glands. In the latter glands, the upper lip is the site of predilection, followed by the buccal mucosa [43]. Patients have been reported with multifocal or bilateral occurrence.

Sialolithiasis in the submandibular gland may or may not cause symptoms, consisting of pain or discomfort before or during meals. Recurrent submandibular swelling is often mentioned. Infection of the gland may also occur.

In the diagnostic procedure, bimanual dorsoventral massage of the affected gland and the excretory duct should be carried out, observing the flow and the clearness of the saliva. When located in the excretory duct, the calculus can often be located by bimanual palpation, which characteristically causes pain.

6.10.5 Radiographic Aspects

When located in the floor of the mouth, an occlusal radiograph may clearly reveal the stone, sometimes showing lamination. When located in the submandibular gland itself, a lateral skull film or orthopantomogram may be helpful in detecting the sialolith. However, in the early stage of calculus formation, the radiographic findings are negative [47]. In such cases, xeroradiography may be a valuable aid [41]. Furthermore, ultrasonographic examination can be very useful. The use of endoscopy as a technique for diagnosis has also been described [74].

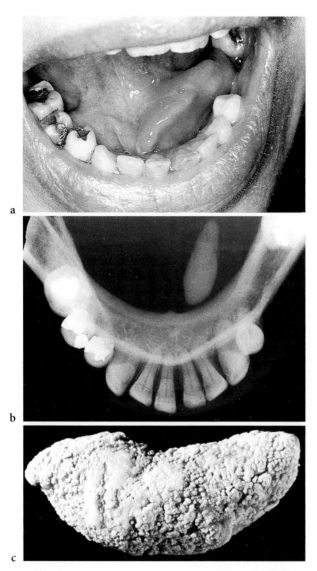

Fig. 6.14. a Unilateral, painful swelling of the floor of the mouth. **b** The occlusal radiograph confirms the tentative diagnosis of a sialolith. **c** The sialolith after removal

Rounded-off structures on a radiograph may also be based on phleboliths, calcified lymph nodes, or a pilomatrixoma of the skin [73]. Sialoliths have a more opaque center than phleboliths or calcified lymph nodes. In some instances, a sialolith in the floor of the mouth is manifest radiographically as an opaque lesion of the mandibular bone (Fig. 6.15).

Sialography may be useful by showing a relative radiolucency or a total blockage in the excretory system (Fig. 6.16). In this procedure, displacement of the calculus toward the gland cannot always be avoided.

There is rarely a need for scintigraphic examination when dealing with a sialolith, since the decision whether or not to remove the submandibular gland itself is usually made on clinical grounds. Furthermore, absence of activity does not rule out the possibility of functional recovery after removal of the stone [3].

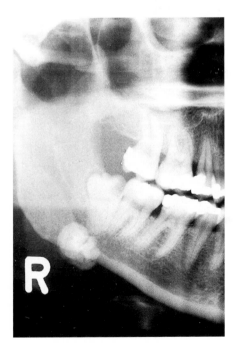

Fig. 6.15. Radiopaque structure near the angle of the mandible based on a sialolith of the submandibular gland

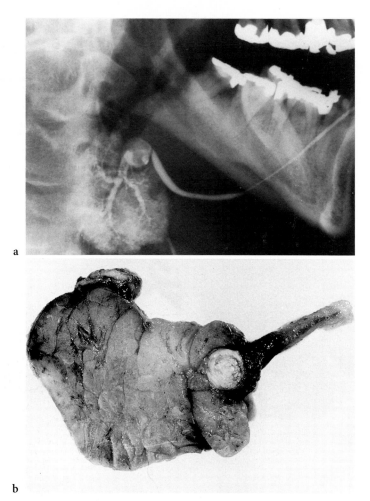

a

b

Fig. 6.16. a Sialogram of patient with a sialolith in the hilum of the submandibular gland. **b** Cross-section of surgical specimen

6.10.6 Treatment

Sialoliths of the excretory duct of the submandibular gland can usually be removed via an intraoral approach, either using local or general anesthesia [87]. When located in the gland itself, extirpation of the gland is often indicated. Some promising papers have been pub-

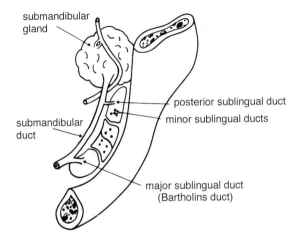

submandibular
gland

submandibular
duct

posterior sublingual duct

minor sublingual ducts

major sublingual duct
(Bartholins duct)

Fig. 6.17. Sublingual
glandular complex,
explaining the
recurrence of sialoliths
in the submandibular
duct. (Reprinted with
permission from [82])

lished on laser lithotripsy [46, 67] and on removal by using salivary gland endoscopy [74].

Calculi in the excretory duct of the parotid gland can usually be removed without great difficulties. Intraparotid stones rarely give rise to serious clinical signs or symptoms. Thus there is actually no indication for parotid surgery in such instances.

Sialoliths of the intraoral salivary glands can be removed by a simple surgical procedure.

Recurrent calculus formation is rare. Such cases have been reported in the submandibular duct many years after the removal of the submandibular gland, presumably due to the existence of communications between the sublingual glandular complex and the remaining submandibular duct (Fig. 6.17) [82]. Occasionally, contralateral sialolithiasis may develop.

Some authors recommend performing a scintigraphic examination after sialolithiasis [109]. However, the absence of activity does not necessarily require removal of the gland.

6.11 Irradiation Damage of Salivary Gland Tissue

In irradiation of head and neck cancer, it is often unavoidable to include one or more of the major salivary glands in the field of irradiation. At a total dose of approximately 20 Gy, severe, yet probably reversible damage of the salivary glands takes place. At higher doses, irreversible changes are induced, consisting of atrophy and eventually fibrosis of the acinar structures. Glands that are partially irradiated are more likely to have some residual function than fully irradiated glands; furthermore, the submandibular and sublingual glands are clearly dysfunctional in postirradiation xerostomia patients compared with controls in terms of both flow rates and sialochemistry [104]. Salivary scintigraphy is a suitable method to assess radiation-induced salivary gland injury. The test is able to detect salivary glandular dysfunction in an early phase and may be useful to predict which patients will respond to salivary stimulants [103].

The cause of the acute effects of radiation on salivary function is not known; these early effects may be due to damage to the blood supply or to the interference with transmission of nerve impulses. The later effects are due to the destruction of the gland's secretory apparatus and its subsequent replacement by fibrous connective tissue and also to specific vascular damage (endarteritis).

The resulting xerostomia is difficult to manage, although early treatment with pilocarpine still may be effective (see Chap. 1). Preliminary results have been reported of the use of bethanechol (25 mg three times daily) [28] and carbacholine, another cholinergic drug [48].

References

1. Abrams AM, Melrose RJ, Howell FV. Necrotizing sialometaplasia. A disease simulating malignancy. Cancer 1973; 32: 130–135.
2. Adam P, Haroun A, Billet J, et al. Biopsie des glandes salivaires. Intérêt et technique de la biopsie de la glande sublinguale sur sont versant antéro-latéral. Rev Stomatol Chir maxillofac 1992; 93: 337–340.
3. Akker van den HP. Diagnostic imaging in salivary gland disease. Oral Surg Oral Med Oral Pathol 1988; 66: 625–637.
4. Anavi Y, Mintz S. Benign lymphoepithelial lesion of the sublingual gland. J Oral Maxillofac Surg 1992; 50: 1111–1113.
5. Atkinson JC, Schi dt M, Robataille S, et al. Salivary autoantibodies in HIV-associated salivary gland disease. J Oral Pathol Med 1993; 22: 203–206.
6. Autio-Harmainen H, Pääkkö P, Alavaikko M, et al. Familial occurrence of malignant lymphoepithelial lesion of the parotid gland in a Finnish family with dominantly inherited trichoepithelioma. Cancer 1988; 61: 161–166.

7. Baddour HM, Ripley JF, Cortex EA, et al. Treatment of Frey's syndrome by an inter-positional fascia graft: report of case. J Oral Surg 1980; 38: 778–781.

8. Barak S, Katz J, Mintz S. Anterior lingual mandibular salivary gland defect – a dilemma in diagnosis. Br J Oral Maxillofac Surg 1993; 31: 318–320.

9. Barrett AW, Speight PM. Adenomatoid hyperplasia of minor salivary glands. Oral Surg Oral Med Oral Pathol 1995; 79: 482–487.

10. Batsakis JG. The pathology of head and neck tumors: the lymphoepithelial lesion and Sjögren's syndrome. Part 16. Head Neck Surg 1982; 5: 150–163.

11. Batsakis JG, Manning JT. Necrotizing sialometaplasia of major salivary glands. J Laryngol Otol 1987; 101: 962–966.

12. Beitler JJ, Vikram B, Silver CE, et al. Low-dose radiotherapy for multicystic benign lymphoepithelial lesions of the parotid gland in HIV-positive patients: long-term results. Head & Neck 1995; 17: 31–35.

13. Ben-Aryeh H, Gordon N, Szargel R, et al. Whole saliva in systemic lupus erythematosus patients. Oral Surg Oral Med Oral Pathol 1993; 75: 696–699.

14. Black MJ, Gunna A. The management of Frey's syndrome with aluminum chloride hexahydrate antiperspirant. Ann R Coll Surg Eng 1990; 72: 49–52.

15. Bosch JD, Kudryk WH, Johnson GH. The malignant lymphoepithelial lesion of the salivary glands. J Otolaryngol 1988; 17: 187–190.

16. Brannon RB, Fowler CB, Hartman KS. Necrotizing sialometaplasia. A clinicopathologic study of sixty-nine cases and review of the literature. Oral Surg Oral Med Oral Pathol 1991; 72: 317–325.

17. Chen CY, Ohba T. An analysis of radiological findings of Stafne's idiopathic bone cavity. Dentomaxillofac Radiol 1981; 10: 18–23.

18. Chomette G, Auriol M, Habib K, et al. Intérêt de la biopsie des glandes salivaires accessoires labiales pour le diagnostic d'amylose. Rev Stomatol Chir maxillofac 1992; 93: 54–57.

19. Cleary KR, Batsakis JG. Lymphoepithelial cysts of the parotid region: A "new face" on an old lesion. Ann Otol Rhinol Laryngol 1990; 99: 162–164. (A).

20. Colebunders R, Francis H, Mann JM, et al. Parotid swelling during human immunodeficiency virus infection. Arch Otolaryngol Head Neck Surg 1988; 114: 330–332.

21. Cook JN, Layton SA. Bilateral parotid swelling associated with chronic obstructive pulmonary disease. A case of pneumoparotid. Oral Surg Oral Med Oral Pathol 1993; 76: 157–158.

22. Danford M. Facial sinus formation secondary to a parotid duct calculus. Br Dent J 1993; 175: 73–74.

23. Dawson Watts K. Congenital imperforate parotid duct openings: a case report. Br J Oral Maxillofac Surg 1988; 26: 341–343.

24. Dean DH, Hiramoto RN. Submandibular salivary gland involvement in hemochromatosis. J Oral Med 1984; 39: 197–198.

25. Di Giusto E, Eckhard I. Some properties of saliva cotinine measurements in indicating exposure to tobacco smoking. Am J Publ Health 1986; 76: 1245–1246.

26. Drobik C, Laskawi R, Schwab S. Die Therapie des Frey-Syndroms mit Botulinumtoxin A. Erfahrungen mit einer neuen Behandlungsmethode. HNO 1995; 43: 644–648.

27. Dubois D, Debeney-Bruyere C, Derbin Y, et al. Aplasie des glandes salivaires principales. A propos d'une observation de xérostomie. Rev Stomatol Chir maxillofac 1994; 95: 118–119.

28. Epstein JB, Burchell JL, Emerton S, et al. A clinical trial of bethanechol in patients with xerostomia after radiation therapy. A pilot study. Oral Surg Oral Med Oral Pathol 1994; 77: 610–614.

29. Falzon M, Isaacson PG. The natural history of benign lymphoepithelial lesion of the salivary gland in which there is a monoclonal population of B cells. A report of two cases. Am J Surg Pathol 1991; 15: 59–65.

30. Faussat J-M, Ghiassi B, Princ G. Une rhinorrhée d'origine parotidienne. A propos d'un cas. Rev Stomatol Chir maxillofac 1993; 94: 363–365.

31. Finfer MD, Schinella RA, Rothstein SG, et al. Cystic parotid lesions in patients at risk for the acquired immunodeficiency syndrome. Arch Otolaryngol Head Neck Surg 1988; 114: 1290–1294.

32. Fishleder A, Tubbs R, Hesse B, et al. Uniform detection of immunoglobulin-gene rearrangement in benign lymphoepithelial lesions. New Engl J Med 1987; 316: 1118–1121.

33. Frerichs RR, Htoon MT, Eskes N, et al. Comparison of saliva and serum for HIV surveillance in developing countries. Lancet 1992; 340: 1496–1499.

34. Goguen LA, April MM, Karmody CS, et al. Self-induced pneumoparotis. Arch Otolaryngol Head Neck Surg 1995; 121: 1426–1429.

35. Goldman RL, Klein HZ. Proliferative sialometaplasia arising in an intraparotid lymph node. Am J Clin Pathol 1986; 86: 116–119.

36. Gombar KK, Singh B. Bilateral parotid sialadenopathy associated with general anesthesia: a case report. J Oral Maxillofac Surg 1993; 51: 328–330.

37. Gordeeff A, Piot B, Gaillard F, et al. Aspects pronostiques et thérapeutiques des lésions lympho-épithéliales de la parotide. A propos de 8 observations. Rev Stomatol Chir maxillofac 1990; 94: 44–48.

38. Grötz KA, Menstell S. Manifestation einer Sialadenose bei psychogener Eßstörung. Dtsch Z Mund Kiefer GesichtsChir 1993; 17: 181–184.

39. Haddock A, Porter SR, Scully C, et al. Submandibular gustatory sweating. Oral Surg Oral Med Oral Pathol 1994; 77: 317.

40. Hasler JF. Parotid enlargement: A presenting sign in anorexia nervosa. Oral Surg Oral Med Oral Pathol 1982; 53: 567–573.

41. Haug RH, Bradrick JP, Thomas Indresano A. Xeroradiography in the diagnosis of nonradiopaque sialoliths. Oral Surg Oral Med Oral Pathol 1989; 67: 146–148.

42. Hays LL. The Frey Syndrome: a review and double blind evaluation of the topical use of a new anticholinergic agent. Laryngoscope 1978; 88: 1796–1824.

43. Ho V, Currie WJR, Walker A. Sialolithiasis of minor salivary glands. Br J Oral Maxillofac Surg 1992; 30: 273–275.

44. Hyjek E, Smith WJ, Isaacson PG. Primary B-cell lymphoma of salivary glands and its relationship to myoepithelal sialadenitis. Hum Pathol 1988; 19: 766–776.

45. Ioachim HL, Ryan JR, Blaugrund SM. Salivary gland lymph nodes. The site of lymphadenopathies and lymphomas associated with human immunodeficiency virus infection. Arch Pathol Lab Med 1988; 112: 1224–1228.

46. Iro H, Benzel W, Zenk J, et al. Minimal-invasive Behandlung der Sialolithiasis mittels extrakorporaler Stoßwellen. HNO 1993; 41: 311–316.

47. Isacsson G, Isberg A, Haverling M, et al. Salivary calculi and chronic sialoadenitis of the submandibular gland: A radiographic and histologic study. Oral Surg Oral Med Oral Pathol 1984; 58: 622–627.

48. Joensuu H, Boström P, Makkonen T. Pilocarpine and carbacholine in treatment of radiation-induced xerostomia. Radiotherapy and Oncology 1993; 26: 33–37.

49. Kabakkaya Y, Dogan M. Bakan E, et al. Bilateral parotid duct fistula. Case report. Ann Otol Rhinol Laryngol 1993; 102: 375–377.

50. Kelly SA, Black MJM, Soames JV. Unilateral enlargement of the parotid gland in a patient with sialosis and contralateral parotid aplasia. Br J Oral Maxillofac Surg 1990; 28: 409–412.

51. Khullar SM, Best PV. Adenomatosis of minor salivary glands. Report of a case. Oral Surg Oral Med Oral Pathol 1992; 74: 783–787.

52. Krishnamurthy S, Lanier AP, Dohan P, et al. Salivary gland cancer in Alaskan natives, 1966–1980. Hum Pathol 1987; 18: 986–996.

53. Kubo S, Abe K, Ureshino T, et al. Aplasia of the submandibular gland. A case report. J Cranio-Max-Fac Surg 1990; 18: 119–121.

54. Laccourreye O, Bonan B, Brasnu D, et al. Treatment of Frey's syndrome with topical 2% diphemanil methylsulfate (Prantal[R]): a double-blind evaluation of 15 patients. Laryngoscope 1990; 100: 651–653.

55. Lamey P-J, Felix D, Nolan A. Case report. Sialectasis and HIV infection. Dentomaxillofac Radiol 1993; 22: 159–160.

56. Langone JJ, Cook G, Bjercke RJ et al. Monoclonal antibody ELISA for cotinine in saliva and urine of active and passive smokers, J Immunol Methods 1988; 114: 73–78.

57. Lustmann J, Regev, Melamed Y. Sialolithiasis. A survey on 245 patients and a review of the literature. Int J Oral Maxillofac Surg 1990; 19: 135–138.

58. Mandel LM, Kaynar A, DeChiara S. Necrotizing sialometaplasia in a patient with sickle-cell anemia. J Oral Maxillofac Surg 1991; 49: 757–759.

59. Mandel LM, Reich R. HIV parotid gland lymhpoepithelial cysts. Review and case reports. Oral Surg Oral Med Oral Pathol 1992; 74: 273–278.

60. Mandel LM, Kaynar A. Bulimia and parotid swelling: a review and case report. J Oral Maxillofac Surg 1992; 50: 1122–1125.

61. Mandel ID. The diagnostic uses of saliva. J Oral Pathol Med 1990; 19: 119–125.

62. Mandel L, Kaynar A. Sialadenopathy: a clinical herald of sarcoidosis: report of two cases. J Oral Maxillofac Surg 1994; 52: 1208–1210.

63. Marchetti P, Grossi C, Giannarelli R, et al. Salivary immunoreactive insulin: a new entry in clinical chemistry? Clin Chem 1988; 34: 1478–1480.

64. Marker P. A case of benign lymphoepithelial lesion of the hard palate. Int J Oral Surg 1983; 12: 348–354.

65. Matthews JB, Potts AJC, Hamburger J, et al. Immunoglobulin-producing cells in labial salivary glands of patients with rheumatoid arthritis and systemic lupus erythematosus. J Oral Pathol 1986; 15: 520–523.

66. May JS, McGuirt WF. Frey's syndrome: treatment with topical glycopyrrolate. Head & Neck 1989; 11: 85–89.

67. McGurk M, Prince MJ, Jiang ZX, et al. Laser lithotripsy: a preliminary study on its application for sialolithiasis. Br J Oral Maxillofac Surg 1994; 32: 218–221.

68. Mealey BL. Bilateral gustatory sweating as a sign of diabetic neuropathy. Oral Surg Oral Med Oral Pathol 1994; 77: 113–115.

69. Mesa ML, Gerber RS, Schneider LC. Necrotizing sialometaplasia: frequency of histologic misdiagnosis. Oral Surg Oral Med Oral Pathol 1984; 57: 71–73.

70. Miller CS, Dembo JB, Falace DA et al. Salivary cortisol response to dental treatment of varying stress. Oral Surg Oral Med Oral Pathol 1995; 79: 436–441.

71. Moody GH. Oral pathology in Papua New Guinea. Int J Oral Maxillofac Surg 1982; 11: 240–245.

72. Murty GE, Mains BT, Bennett MK. Salivary gland involvement in Wegener's granulomatosis. J Laryngol Otol 1990; 104: 259–261.

73. Muto T, Michiya H, Kanazawa M, et al. Pathological calcification of the cervico-facial region. Br J Oral Maxillofac Surg 1991; 29: 120–122.

74. Nahlieli O, Neder A, Baruchin AM. Salivary gland endoscopy: a new technique for diagnosis and treatment of sialolithiasis. J Oral Maxillofac Surg 1994; 52: 1240–1242.

75. Nash M, Cho H, Cohen J. Salivary choristomas in the neck. Otolaryngol Head Neck Surg 1988; 99: 590–593.

76. Nessan VJ, Jacoway JR. Biopsy of minor salivary glands in the diagnosis of sarcoidosis. N Engl J Med 1979; 301: 922–924.

77. O'Malley AM, Macleod RI, Welbury RR. Congenital aplasia of major salivary glands in a 4-year-old child. International Journal of Paediatric Dentistry 1993; 3: 141–144.

78. Ogren FP, Huerter JV, Pearson PH, et al. Transient salivary gland hypertrophy in bulimics. Laryngoscope 1987; 97: 951–953.

79. Ohishi K, Ueno R, Nishino S, et al. Increased level of salivary prostaglandins in patients with major depression. Biol Psychiatry 1988; 23: 326–334.

80. Ott KHR. Die Messung der Quecksilber-Belastung im Speichel. Dtsch Zahnärztl Z 1993; 48: 154–157.

81. Palmer RM, Eveson JW, Gusterson BA. "Epimyoepithelial" islands in lymphoepithelial lesions. An immunocytochemical study. Virchows Archiv [Pathol Anat] 1986; 408: 603–609.

82. Patton DW. Recurrent calculus formation following removal of the subman-dibular salivary gland. Br J Oral Maxillofac Surg 1987; 25: 15–20.

83. Petri WH, Carr RF, Kahn CS. Adenomatoid hyperplasia of the palate. J Oral Maxillofac Surg 1993; 51: 310–311.

84. Piette E, Walker RT. Pneumoparotid during dental treatment. Oral Surg Oral Med Oral Pathol 1991; 72: 415–417.

85. Poulson TC, Greer RO, Ryser RW. Necrotizing sialometaplasia obscuring an underlying malignancy: report of a case. J Oral Maxillofac Surg 1984; 44: 570–574.

86. Redleaf MI, Bauer CA, Robinson RA. Fine-needle detection of cytomegalovirus parotitis in a patient with acquired immunodeficiency syndrome. Arch Otolaryngol Head Neck Surg 1994; 120: 414–416.

87. Rontal M, Rontal E. The use of sialodochoplasty in the treatment of benign inflammatory obstructive submandibular gland disease. Laryngoscope 1987; 97: 1417–1421.

88. Schi dt M, Dodd CL, Greenspan D, et al. Natural history of HIV-associated salivary gland disease. Oral Surg Oral Med Oral Pathol 1992; 74: 326–331.

89. Schmelzer A, Rosin V, Steinbach E. Zur Therapie des Freyschen Syndroms durch ein Anhidrotische Gel. Laryngo-Rhino-Otol 1992; 71: 59–63.

90. Schnitt SJ, Antonioli DA, Jaffe B, et al. Granulomatous inflammation of minor salivary gland ducts: a new oral manifestation of Crohn's disease. Human Pathol 1987; 18: 405–407.

91. Scott J, Burns J, Flower EA. Histological analysis of parotid and submandibular glands in chronic alcohol abuse: a necropsy study. J Clin Pathol 1988; 41: 837–840.

92. Scully C, Davies R, Porter S, et al. HIV-salivary gland disease. Salivary scintiscanning with technetium pertechnetate. Oral Surg Oral Med Oral Pathol 1993; 76: 120–123.

93. Seifert G. WHO International Histological Classification of Tumours. Histological Typing of Salivary Gland Tumours. 2nd ed. Springer-Verlag; Berlin, Heidelberg, New York, 1991.

94. Shugar JMA, Som PM, Jacobson AL, et al. Multicentric parotid cysts and cervical adenopathy in AIDS patients. A newly recognized entity: CT and MR manifestations. Laryngoscope 1988; 98: 772–775.

95. Singh B and Shaha A. Traumatic submandibular salivary gland fistula. J Oral Maxillofac Surg 1995; 53: 338–339.

96. Smith NM, Telfer SM, Byard RW. A comparison of the incidence of cytomegalovirus inclusion bodies in submandibular and tracheobronchial glands in sids and non-sids autopsies. Pediatric Pathology 1992; 12: 185–190.

97. Smith FB, Rajdeo H, Panesar N, et al. Benign lymphoepithelial lesion of the parotid gland in intravenous drug users. Arch Pathol Lab Med 1988; 112: 742–745.

98. Stimson PG, Tortoledo ME, Luna MA, et al. Localized primary amyloid tumor of the parotid gland. Oral Surg Oral Med Oral Pathol 1988; 66: 466–469.

99. Takenoshita Y, Kawano Y, Oka M. Pneumoparotis, an unusual occurrence of parotid gland swelling during dental treament. Report of a case with a review of the literature. J Cranio-Max-Fac Surg 1991; 19: 362–365.

100. Taxy JB. Necrotizing squamous/mucinous metaplasia in oncocytic salivary gland tumors. A potential diagnostic problem. Am J Clin Pathol 1992; 97: 40–45.

101. Tunkel DE, Loury MC, Fox CH, et al. Bilateral parotid enlargement in HIV-seropositive patients. Laryngoscope 1989; 99: 590–595.

102. Urquia M, Rodriguez-Archilla A, Gonzalez-Moles MA, et al. Detection of anti-HIV antibodies in saliva. J Oral Pathol Med 1993; 22: 153–156.

103. Valdés Ormos RA, Keus RB, Takes RP, et al. Scintigraphic assessment of salivary function and excretion response in radiation-induced injury of the major salivary glands. Cancer 1994; 73: 2886–2893.

104. Valdez IH, Atkinson JC, Ship JA, et al. Major salivary gland function in patients with radiation-induced xerostomia: flow rates and sialochemistry. Int J Radiation Oncology Biol Phys 1993; 25: 41–47.
105. Vijay V, Newman R, Bebawi MA, et al. Sarcoid ranula. Its assocation with widespread sarcoidosis. Oral Surg Oral Med Oral Pathol 1995; 79: 449–451.
106. Wal van der JE, Waal van der I. Necrotizing sialometaplasia: report of 12 new cases. Br J Oral Maxillofac 1990; Surg 28: 326–328.
107. Waterhouse JP, Chisholm DM, Winter RB, et al. Replacement of functional parenchymal cells by fat and connective tissue in human submandibular glands: An age-related change. J Oral Pathol 1973; 2: 16–27.
108. Wiesenfeld D, Iverson ES, Ferguson MM, et al. Familial parotid gland aplasia. J Oral Med 1985; 40: 84–85.
109. Yoshimura Y, Morishita T, Sugihara T. Salivary gland function after sialolithiasis: scintigraphic examination of submandibular glands with [99m]TcPertechnetate. J Oral Maxillofac Surg 1989; 47: 704–710.

Subject Index

Springer-Verlag
and the Environment

We at Springer-Verlag firmly believe that an international science publisher has a special obligation to the environment, and our corporate policies consistently reflect this conviction.

We also expect our business partners – paper mills, printers, packaging manufacturers, etc. – to commit themselves to using environmentally friendly materials and production processes.

The paper in this book is made from low- or no-chlorine pulp and is acid free, in conformance with international standards for paper permanency.

Printing: Druckerei Stolinski, Malsch
Binding: Buchbinderei Schäffer, Grünstadt